RICH TRAINER, POOR TRAINER

Copyright 2012 by FreeWill Press

Printed June 2012
Cover Design by Greg Ryan
Editing by Resolutions Publishing
ISBN-13: 978-1467985161

About the Author

At age 46, Greg Ryan, a native of St. Joseph, Michigan, has amassed a striking list of credentials. Beginning at age sixteen, Greg, over a span of thirty years, has accomplished everything one could imagine in the health and fitness industry, and specifically the personal training profession.

In 1990 Greg moved to Los Angeles, California, where his knowledge, enthusiasm and skill attracted the attention of fitness guru Kathy Smith. During this time, Greg ran one of the largest personal training businesses in L.A., attracting numerous high-profile movie stars. Greg built a reputation for exercise and behavior change, and in the fall of 1992 appeared on the *Today Show* and *Good Morning America*.

Greg produced his own television segment on FOX TV in the mid-1990s while attending physical therapy school. In 1997 Greg relocated to Louisville, Kentucky, where he operated a flourishing private clinic specializing in obesity, diabetes and weight loss programs.

In the fall of 2004, Greg authored and published his first of a total of twenty-four books to date on fitness, personal training, body building, steroids and disease. As it relates to *RICH TRAINER, POOR TRAINER*, over the last thirty years Greg has acquired nearly one hundred thousand hours of paid personal training sessions and has designed and helped build a dozen or more training facilities. In that time, he has learned some of the best-kept secrets to being successful as a fitness trainer in both good and bad economic times.

About the Book

RICH TRAINER, POOR TRAINER IS ABOUT THE MINDSET OF CREATING WEALTH.

Not all of you are ready for it, honestly. Some will disregard a lot of it, and only a handful will finish it. Those who finish it are the people who will become wealthy, not because I have the answers, but because of the mindset YOU have. The rest will wish they were and resent the ones who are wealthy.

Why should you read this book?

Every personal trainer who has NOT made a million dollars needs to read *RICH TRAINER, POOR TRAINER*. This series gives you real-life proven formulas for success and building wealth as a fitness trainer. Be careful, though—it may be too simple to comprehend.

From the Author

Whether you think you can or cannot, the outcome will be just that. You get what you believe: self-worth and financial worth. I was just naive enough to think I was worthy of both. With that mindset, four lines on a piece of paper and three decades later, I am about to share with you what to me is priceless!

Making a million bucks as a fitness trainer is NOT all about numbers on a chart or molecular structures you learn in a classroom. Wealth as a fitness trainer is found not in competing, but creating, not from complaining, but gratifying, not from complacency, but consistency.

By all means, get your education; it's part of a good foundation. In the end, however, it comes down to *leadership, common sense, psychology of people and you*. How you relate, motivate, educate, and encourage will make a huge difference; however, by themselves you will not find prosperity or peace within yourself—or the fitness training profession as a whole, for that matter.

I have made millions not for my brains, but for my smarts, not for my ability to design the *"secret"* exercise program, but for my keen awareness of how one should think. Not with the sharpest of minds in a classroom, I will admit, but creativity, intuition and the ability to feel things into existence through faith, common sense and will—I'll say there may not be any better. But really I'm just a common person who had a dream that never died, humble enough to admit imperfections, and the willingness to work smart through thought and the wisdom of others rather than ego. Just being *"open-minded"* will separate you from most. However......

A word of caution!

Be extremely careful not to make the mistakes most fitness trainers make. Making money is not complicated. However, hardly any do, and why is that? Heck, most of you won't even read this entire intro, let alone the whole book. If you fail to do even that, how in the world do you expect to be successful, forget being wealthy...

If you get into personal training for the glamour, get out NOW; "glamour" meaning for the fun of it. You won't last anyway; the business will spit you out like a scalding sip of coffee. And yes, it is a *business*. In the end, all you will do is cast a bad, unprofessional light on the industry. The fitness training industry is in desperate need of business-minded people, career-oriented individuals—*"lifers,"* if you will.

RICH TRAINER, POOR TRAINER is a two hundred eighty-page book that outlines key areas of thinking and what it takes to be a successful fitness trainer; it gives hundreds of ideas and experiences learned on the job, not in the classroom. Just one piece of advice could double or triple your income; if, and only if, you are willing to follow through with your dreams. This series outlines the one biggest **secret** to becoming **financially** independent as a fitness **trainer.**

The sad thing is that ninety percent of you reading this right now will give up on your dreams, because you were either too egotistical to learn or fail to think beyond your imagination. I will be the first to tell you, I don't claim to have all the answers, but I have learned a whole heck of a lot in thirty years, and have sustained a great cash flow in good and bad economic times. My father taught me that if you want to have what others have, then learn and listen to them first, and ask question second.

I want to challenge you RIGHT NOW to get serious about your future, but I ask of you one thing: Swallow your pride. There's no other single thing that costs trainers more money than this! But, who am I to say such a thing?

Who is Greg Ryan?

Well, there was a time growing up when I wasn't sure. I was not a confident dude, nor did I have the slightest idea the direction my life would take. Raised on a farm with a work ethic out of necessity, God saw something. What in the world could he do with an introverted, unmotivated medium-educated boy from a small town in Michigan?

Well, fitness found me and personally changed it all— probably more like he unlocked the key to the real guy inside; fitness was just the vehicle to better things.

5

How did it all happen?

The beginning was just a blur; it was challenging just to ride the wave. First, the opportunity to compete as a bodybuilder was completely different than anything I had done or had the personality for. Following that up with finding myself in a well-respected leadership role of coaching others on fitness was, at the time, almost laughable, besides the fact of making money at it.

How did I get into fitness training? *"Accidental coincidences,"* I say. Fitness found me, and I found a career. Four lines on a piece of paper and three decades later, here I am.

Maybe I was just at the right place at the right time in my life? I don't know. Maybe it was accidentally walking through the wrong door at college, where I met two of what ended up being the greatest friends and support I could ever have? Or maybe it was truly those four lines I wrote on that scrap paper as a teenager that read:

"Only by the Grace of God in America

could one get paid, be prosperous and live their dream,

by teaching people to strive for healthy lives through exercise.

LORD, let that be me."

Looking back, maybe it was just me being naive enough to believe those words that put me in the car that day. Oh, that day, I remember it well: August 17, 1989. With five hundred dollars to my name, no job or direction, holding just a hope in my heart and a dream in my mind, I left the world only as I knew it, in search of a what? I was not sure. What I am sure of is that there are no coincidences in life, no accidental circumstances that just happen to find you. We all have our place in this life to touch just the right person at the most

—

appropriate time. How did it all happen? I'm not sure how, but I do know why.

Why have I stayed?

I have stayed because of how it all happened. I have stayed in the fitness business because of the promise I made to myself and those that I am yet to have met. The day I left for California, I decided that fitness training was my calling, the very thing that I was born to do. It had changed my life, saved it no less, and now through me I must help change another. I have stayed thirty years due to that promise and because I have yet to meet the one for the very reason it has all started in the first place.

What is RICH TRAINER, POOR TRAINER?

My life, I guess you could say. This book series is an accumulation of my experiences, trials, tribulations, mistakes and triumphs that I would not change for all the money in the world. *RICH TRAINER, POOR TRAINER* is to me one of the only and most important ways I could ever give back to the industry what it has given me: knowledge, wisdom, gratification, courage, belief and even peace.

What is *RICH TRAINER, POOR TRAINER?* Priceless, in my opinion. And it is my prayer that if you are serious about the fitness training profession, you too will decide to read it.

Sincerely Yours,

Greg Ryan

FREE Your Mind!

Content

Personality Type Programming- *One Size Fits NOT All*
Storytelling for Cash- *Reality, Relativity and Repetition*

Leadership 101- *The "Purpose" of the Plan*
Lead with Confidence- *Believe or Be Left Behind*
Lead with Love- *The Truth Will Set You Free*
Lead with Silence- *Stillness Breeds Knowledge*
Lead with Boundaries- *Structuring for Success*
Lead with Accountability- *Empowerment through Responsibility*

Marketing 101- *The "Power" through Brand Leverage*
Branding You- *Repeat Business through Remembrance*
The Pied Piper Principle- *The Money Is in the List*
Leveraging Your Brand- *The Power of Duplication*
Synergizing the Social Media Wave- *Momentum makes Money Fast*

Nutrition 101 – *The "Influence" of the Role Play*
The Goal- *Know Your Plan Ahead of Time*
The Role Player- *Knowing Your Place*
The Big Picture Painting- *It's an Attitude*
The Pen Power- *The Power behind the Awareness*
The Programming for Personality- *The Approach*

BONUS MATERIAL
Gym and Fitness Director 101 – *The "Magic" of Profit*
Gym Owners- Profit Margins- *Retention, Reliable, and Real Good* Trainers- *Win-Win*
Trainer Dude 100
100 Things I Did Not Learn in the Classroom

COMING IN OCTOBER- NEW BOOK!

The "Art" Of Fitness Training- *An Old School Approach with a New School Look!* Secrets to Success behind the Numbers on the Charts! Go to www.rich-trainer for book preview.

RICH TRAINER, POOR TRAINER

Mission Statement- To evaluate and educate trainers, coaches, gym owners or any fitness professional of certain *"mindsets"* on how to build wealth and enjoy a successful fitness career.

Goal- To help fitness experts understand the little secrets to business, marketing, people skills, psychology, and leadership of the fitness training industry.

Five-Year Plan- Full-time book publisher, educator and speaker!

Vision- Worldwide educator on *"wealth-building in fitness"*!

Promise- To give the world the most realistic, common-sense, truthful knowledge of what it takes to be the best trainer one can be. To not get above reproach or lose sight of the main thing—this I promise.

Do not make your profession in the fitness world complicated; it's not. Don't think that you have arrived at any point in your career, because that will be the beginning of the end for you. Do, however, compete only with yourself. Fuel the creativity inside; never fall prey to small-minded thinking on the outside, and love people for who they are, not what you want them to become.

Greg Ryan

Introduction

You get what you think and give. You attract into your business what you believe to be your truth, maybe not even the reality of the moment; this is a scary game one must not play, whatever your goals are in life. It's the little things that make the big differences. Pay attention to detail, yet manage from afar.

Greg Ryan

Introduction

A word to the wise! This book may not be what you are expecting. The information within these pages is not so much about X's and O's as it is about your **"mindset"** behind them.

The fact is that the majority of fitness trainers will fail—not because they do not have enough education, but because they have no idea of what it takes to be successful in the industry. Being a mediocre trainer is not complicated; being a RICH one is even easier if you know what to focus on. It's not what you think it is, either.

Joe the Millionaire

Average Joe becomes a millionaire not because he's lucky; he becomes wealthy because of how he thinks, more so than what he does. Joe also knows that becoming RICH is more about doing less, more effectively. RICH people make money regardless of the state of the economy. They make no excuses or entertain a victim mentality, nor do they try to reinvent something that already makes them money.

They purposely find people who have what they want, and mirror their habits. In other words, they find the rivers of money and ride the wave all the way to the bank.

*Joe the **Rich** Trainer*

Making a million as a trainer is no different; observe poor ones, and then do mostly the opposite. Seek out trainers making money, and get to know them.

Again, getting RICH as a trainer is not about exercise charts; it's about how you think and not breaking what's NOT broken. If you want to be wealthy, do what the wealthy trainers are doing. If you don't, then you will be....

*Joe the **Poor** Trainer*

Joe the poor trainer does everything his way. Denial, ego and pride strips him of wealth without him even realizing it. He spends tons of money on gimmicky ads and neglects the true moneymaking principles; in short, Joe the *Poor* trainer is lazy, egotistical, small-minded and inconsistent. He or she is a loner, full of fear, and at the core feels that he is not worthy to be wealthy, especially if it's possible to do it doing something he loves to do.

Wealth is acquired first in your head, then in your wallet. The main question is: **"Do you feel you deserve it?"** Seriously, think about this! If you are not making the money you want, then deep down, you don't deserve it, or so you think. But, Joe the Millionaire does, so he THINKS.

Joe Knows

Joe lives in a small town, big town, next door, up the road or across street. Joe doesn't care where he resides or what others think; he just knows. He knows most will fail while he succeeds. He knows he will listen to wise counsel when others won't. He knows you don't have to be special to do great things. Joe knows how to be wealthy before he sees cash, but most of all, Joe knows that you can be him if you realize that money and wealth come not from charts or graphs, but from something else.

I
The "X" Factor

The "Secret" to Cash

This book is about how I took a treadmill, row of dumbbells, stretching mat and a dream and made my first million dollars.

Greg Ryan

1
The "X" Factor

Why do some people end up successful and others do not? You can have two different people who do the exact thing in a business or career and have totally opposite outcomes. Is one person just luckier than the other? Are the richer people smarter than the rest? Or do the wealthy know something that most do not? Those answers may surprise you.

A RICH fitness trainer and a POOR one are separated by really two things: **how they think, and how they use what God has given them.** Sounds simple, but if that were the case, why are there not more successful fitness trainers or coaches?

"How have you been able to stay in the business of personal training, let alone be very successful at it?" many will ask.

You have got to have something *extra*. RICH trainers first have a quality that cannot be taught. I call it **the "X" Factor.** In other words, you need to have the talents of a Simon Cowell in fitness.

The Gift

I am all for education and certifications. God knows, I have spent a few hours with my nose in a book. However to be successful as a fitness trainer it takes more, it takes something special. It takes a combination of *people skills, psychology, common sense, leadership, confidence and mindset,* all summed up into something that cannot be explained.

A "gift" can be anything. The word *gift* just describes something given to you. What's unique about a gift is the value you put on it; only you can decide that. The same gift given to one may mean nothing, but to you it's priceless and words could not describe it.

While the information in this book series to me is worth a million dollars, to you it may only be worth the money you pay for the book. With most, you only get what you put into it. So I hope you take these words to heart. So, *"Why do you think few fitness trainers succeed when most do not?"*

The first answer lies in your gift; the second is in what you do best; at the end of the day, you either have it or you don't. I can teach you the business and the smart way of making money as a fitness trainer, but I cannot give you the "X" factor. This should not discourage you. Your talents can and will be found if you *"will"* them to.

I can share many examples of fitness trainers who one day just seemed to get it; they discovered a new part of them that made all the difference in the world. They say:

"When the teacher is ready, the student appears."

I didn't think I had it or even knew what "X" was, but I did have a great attitude. For whatever reason, though, one day if I kept at it, something would click. Having the *"Just one day at a time"* mindset allowed me to stay with it just long enough to see my labors bear fruit, more fruit and even more fruit. Even if you are so-called *"gifted"* or have a special talent, that alone will not guarantee a smooth ride to wealth in the fitness industry. You have got to have something else to go along with it.

The "IT" Factor

While the **"X"** factor has to do with you and your mindset, there's another component to wealth in fitness, what I call *The "IT" Factor.* People, common sense, psychology, business, leadership, nutrition, and marketing make up the second piece to success as a fitness trainer.

While I cannot guarantee you finding <u>"X,"</u> or following through with <u>"IT,"</u> I can outline for you things that worked for me. Do I know all there is to know? No way! But I have learned the hard way how to make continuous money as a fitness trainer for thirty years when most couldn't even survive. Today I have **"IT,"** and would like to share that with you. Tomorrow, you and you alone must discover **"X."**

Let me sum it up by saying this:

"Please, do not make this profession complicated; it's not. Don't think that you have arrived at any point in your career, either, because that will be the beginning of the end for you. Do, however, compete only with yourself, fuel the creativity inside, never fall prey to small-minded thinking, and love people first."

Now, let's get started.

The "X" Factor Review

When you know, that you know, that you know! A gut feeling I guess; you've got to have it. You don't know where or when; you just know you've got it. I can't explain it, pinpoint it, but you know it when it's there; you just get it!

Attitude- You have it or you don't.
Theme- Realize it, nurture it and never take it for granted.
Tagline- The "Secret" to Cash

II
Business 101
The "Foundation" of Wealth

It's not about you, when it comes to the success of your <u>clients.</u> *It IS all about you* when it comes to the success of your <u>business.</u>

Greg Ryan

Business 101 Overview

With any profession or business, there are important elements one must include and build upon in order to be successful long-term. The fitness training *"business,"* is no different.

Attitudes, philosophies, principles, structure, policies and goals all must be part of the developmental planning of your career, from start to finish. If you fail to do so, you will all but guarantee to be added to the ninety percent of fitness trainers who give up on their dreams.

"With no vision, people parish!"

Gaining wealth as a trainer is not complicated. Yes, it's a business, so treat it as such. Find a mentor, and learn the mindset behind any business. **Putting money in your pocket is more of an attitude than writing out exercise programs.**

It's not about you when it comes to the success of your <u>clients.</u> *It IS all about you* when it comes to the success of your <u>business.</u>

Greg Ryan

Attitude Is Everything!

2
It's an Attitude- "Sold Out"

Yes, it's personal! Your career starts with an attitude—not of arrogance, but mindset. The foundation to wealth as a fitness trainer lies in this philosophy that must never be forgotten. You can have the best business principles, practices, goals and aspirations, but at the core, you must be *"Sold Out."*

Sold Out

The only way—and I mean the *only* way—to become successful or RICH as a fitness trainer is to possess an attitude of being "ALL IN," right from the start.

All In

There is a huge difference between a job and a career. When I meet with trainers, I might not ever say a thing, but I know immediately if they are *"All In"* or not. Frankly, ninety percent of you aren't but think you are, and some of you don't even have a clue what I am talking about here.

Most will bail on dreams when the going gets tough, and you can count on it being challenging at times. A heartfelt decision must be made before you even begin: *"Are you in for life or not?"*

Goals Change; Decisions Don't

Before I started my career, I made a quality decision that while my life and goals may change over my lifetime, the decision to be a fitness expert in some way would not. That day, a light came on and never has been turned off.

Flip the Switch Equals Success

I became a professional bodybuilder at a very young age. I became successful not just because of the physical training or even the strange, strict eating habits. I won because of my decision-making ability before I even decided to compete.

I competed once a year and was never a trophy hunter. Each contest required a massive amount of time, energy and dedication. I developed the attitude that if I made a decision I could not turn back, no matter how hard the path would become. In essence, I flipped a switch in my head to not look back. While the goals had to be flexible, the decision was not.

Lifers

The military calls them *"Lifers."* Lifers are individuals who are SOLD OUT to their cause or act of service. There's a much different mindset between a job and a career. Are you a part-time worker or a lifer? Your answer will make the difference between a RICH TRAINER and a POOR TRAINER.

Part-Timer

Trainer jobs are a dime a dozen even in bad economic times. Jobs are for part-time thinkers; jobs are for those who just want to get by in life. If you want to have just a job, that's fine; just don't expect any huge rewards or freedoms that go with it. Yes, you must pay your dues, and you may have to start out having a job, but what I am saying is that part-time attitudes only bring part-time money.

Career

A graduate today will change careers, not jobs, an average of eight times over a lifetime. Career-minded people are more long-term thinkers. Having a career mindset will get you through a *few* of the tough times, but not all. So, what will?

Just one

Keeping a *sold out* attitude is challenging over a prolonged period of time. Years ago, I had to come up with something to get me through the tough times. I had to shorten my goals down to a single day. Each morning, I just thought to myself, *"Oh, just allow me to get through this one day."* All I wanted was one day of a good attitude, thriving business and reaching out to someone to drive in more business. There were many times when I just couldn't think more long-term than just that one day.

Money Tip- You are the extension of your business. The world can tell if you are serious or not. If you are convinced to be a lifer, then the world will bring people into your life. Sounds crazy, but it's true!

Moneymakers flip a switch and never look back.

Your wealth-building ability comes down to how "professional" you are as a fitness trainer and what side of pride you fall on.

Greg Ryan

3
Professional Pride

Yes, it's a business! Sold-out, career-oriented and one-day-at-a-time attitude — now the money will just start rolling in, right? Not so fast. Even if it did, you wouldn't know what to do with it. Before you make your first dollar, you must decide how serious you are going to take the fitness training *profession*. **If you do not learn anything else from this book, remember what you just read: "It's a business!"**

Professional Pride

A sold-out mindset is the key to longevity in a career, but it takes much more than that to become successful in any profession, especially as a fitness trainer. You must have pride in what you are doing, no matter what. Your wealth-building ability comes down to how **"professional"** you are as a fitness trainer and what side of pride you fall on.

Good vs. Bad Pride

There are two types of pride: one that can empower, and one that will destroy you in the end.

The Bad

Bad or negative pride- a high or inordinate opinion of one's own dignity, importance, merit, or superiority, whether as cherished in the mind or as displayed in conduct. *Ego is the root of all poverty.*

This type of pride will cost you a lot of money!

If you ever find yourself above your business or prideful and egotistical, you will also find yourself poor. The fitness business is full of egos and trainers that think they know it all. They are poor not only financially, but emotionally. Pride is always before the fall.

Good Pride

Good Pride is pleasure or satisfaction taken in something done by or belonging to oneself or believed to reflect credit upon oneself—civic pride.

The opposite of bad pride is taking satisfaction in something in helping your clients. If you take good pride in what you are doing, it's almost impossible to not be a professional.

Professionalism

Being a professional at something goes deeper than just knowing your craft. If you want to create wealth as a trainer, you must always maintain and convey these three characteristics; competence, performance and conduct.

Competence

Have sufficient skills or education. In this profession, you see it all. Many are not competent, but have great bodies. Sooner of later, your incompetence will bite you in the butt, because your body will fail you in the end.

Performance

Performance, by definition, means accomplishments against a certain set of standards. Unfortunately, there are no sets of standards in the profession. Performance is NOT just results-oriented either. Performance is a day-to-day striving of "excellence."

Conduct

A standard of behavior best describes what conduct means. This is where trainers fall short. Poor trainers never set standards for themselves; RICH ones do. Set a code of conduct for yourself, and watch how your professionalism soars.

Love It, Respect It or Leave It

In any career or profession, there are things you must understand to survive. If you're not happy doing what you do, all the money in the world won't matter in the end. If you are not mindful of your actions and not treating the profession seriously, you will do it a disservice.

Love It or Leave It

Before I even decided to have a career in fitness, I made a promise to myself to never do something I didn't love. Little did I know that having that sort of attitude would get me through some very tough times. My advice to you is: *"If you don't love it, leave it!"* It's not worth it. In the beginning, this attitude will get you through the tough times, because money will be scarce. If you become a trainer for just a job, you will not survive.

Respect It

One of the biggest reasons the fitness profession as a whole is where it is, is because most trainers do not *"respect"* it. How can you believe in what you do if, deep down, you don't think much of it? How will your business grow if you don't treat it respectfully? You or the business will not reach full potential if you don't fear it in some way. Respect it or leave it!

Perception Is Reality

Why is loving and respecting what you do so important? You cannot expect others to take you seriously if you don't, and you definitely cannot expect people to fork out big bucks, either. People know if you are not in it to win it!

Dress for Success

A trainer came into my office a few weeks back and spent an hour. I told him to come prepared, not waste my or his time and his three hundred dollars. Twenty years ago, I may not have said that, but looking back, I sure wish I had. I'm not sure if he was open to learning anything, but the last thing I said was, *"Tuck your shirt in!"*

The dude paid three hundred dollars for me to tell him to tuck in his shirt. To you that may sound ridiculous, but if you listen, it will make you thousands of dollars. If you get what I am saying, then you are on your way. Professionalism comes in all forms, and can project without even saying a word.

Over time, a majority of fitness trainers have cast a bad light on the profession itself by not taking it seriously.

Life can be about perception. How you look and feel about your profession will determine how others view you and the industry as a whole. Truthfully, a client's success may come down to how seriously they take your advice according to how you are dressed.

If you don't believe me, take college football, for example. Schools spend millions of dollars on uniforms, and why? Studies show that players play better when they feel better, and dressing cool makes them feel better. The investment of the school makes them lots of cash by putting butts in the seats. It's not all about how you dress, but it is all about your competency, performance and conduct. Don't leave money on the table by not being a professional.

Money Tip- Treat your business with the utmost professionalism. Do not get above it by taking anything for granted or acting like you know it all. Love what you do, and the money will follow. The way you feel about your business, all the way down to your dress, will determine how much money you make.

With FREEDOM, how can a price be determined?

4
The Price of Freedom

Yes, it's about freedom! Planning your future is vital to your success. If you are serious about this career and you've decided to treat it like a business then the next step is to develop a five-to-ten-year plan. I realized, at least in the beginning, that I had to pay my dues by getting experience in different environments. However, it just was not in me to work for someone. I wanted to control my own destiny and have the freedom to make my own choices.

What does being FREE mean to you?

Have you ever even thought about what it would be like to have more freedom to do whatever you wanted? What would it be like to be your own boss, call your own shots and even, like myself, go do whatever you wanted, when you wanted, and still get paid? There is no price you can put on that type of living, yet before you get there, there is a price that has to be paid.

The Price of Freedom

With most things in life there are trade-offs, and being out on your own as a trainer is no different. In any career, one will never start out at the top; even if you inherit some sort of business, you will go through growing pains. Another person has controlled my future only four years in my thirty years as a trainer.

Whatever your plan is, a decision should be made sooner rather than later: Let someone control how much you are worth, or control your own life. Not everyone is cut out for either side of that decision. There is a price you will have to pay for having your freedom. The question is: *"How much is that freedom worth to you?"*

Planning for Freedom

Why are you a fitness trainer? Seriously, why are you doing this? Money, fame, status, or how about FREEDOM? Do you know where you will be in five years as a fitness trainer? Do you even know what you want to be doing a few days from now?

The Mission

The hardest thing for any person or company to do is to create a no-more-than-three-sentence-paragraph of their lives and business intentions. Do you have one? If you don't, you will not be wealthy. A mission statement is the very cement that everything else is built off of. The other is your plan.

The Five-Year Business Plan

You want money, plan for it. You want status or fame, plan that, too. While those are superficial at best, at least have a plan to get there. If you want to be free to do whatever you wish and call your own shots, plan for that day. I cannot stress enough the importance of writing out your future plans. A house cannot stand in the long term if a plan is not drawn out first. Not doing a business plan screams:

"YOU ARE NOT SERIOUS!"

Four Lines and a Life Changed Forever

"Only by the Grace of God in America could one get paid to exercise with people, be prosperous doing it while living out one's dream with the goal of teaching people to strive for healthy lives through exercise. LORD, let that be me."

As I sat in my architectural office in 1989, I wrote those words down on a piece of paper. Little did I know that because of them, my life had been put in motion that very moment of writing those words. Six months later almost to the very day, I drove into Los Angeles, California, searching for that dream.

In a few months' time, not knowing WHY, I left my family, fiancée and future back in that small town in Michigan. I had promised myself a few years back that I would not ever do anything I did not LOVE. I wanted to be FREE, and now I am.

Money Tip- If you want to be rich, plan for freedom. There will be a price to pay, but in the end, the rewards are priceless. Freedom gives you the right to control your future. That's money in the bank. However, you will not get to the bank without a map or plan and a car or mission statement. If you don't have one or either, you will continue being poor! If you don't believe me, read Oprah Winfrey's life story.

Change or be changed!

5
Oprah Knows Best

Yes, it's about control! We live in the best country in the world. If you can dream it, you can do it. If you can imagine it, you can make it. I tell people all the time, *"Only in America can a person get paid for working out with people, and in my case paid well."*

Sooner or later you must make a decision that could make the entire difference in your career and, more importantly, your life.

Oprah Knows Best

My father had only a seventh-grade education, yet never had a boss or owed a penny to anyone. He showed me firsthand the benefits of controlling your future and not someone else doing it; Oprah Winfrey was another.

Take Control of Your Life

Oprah decided early in her career that she wanted full control over her life. And frankly, at that time being a female and African-American didn't make it any easy to do so, either. Oprah herself, more than anyone, understood that the decision to go at it alone would bring added stress, scrutiny and self-evaluation; she also believed that it would bring FREEDOM. And that's what America is all about.

I'm sure she has questioned her early decision over time; my dad has, and so have I. But what I have learned—and I am sure they have also—was that the benefits of having FREEDOM are worth every single stressful, uncertain and unpredictable moment.

Having total control over your career is one of the greatest gifts life could ever allow you to experience, and we all have that opportunity.

My dad and Oprah new what was best for them. I learned that too, and now encourage you to think about it, as well. Sooner rather than later, you need to make a decision: Work for yourself, or continue to give your life to another. So in the end, it's better to take the Oprah approach: have the ability and flexibility to explore all your options all the time.

Self-Employed vs. Gym Rat

If you have not made this decision, one day you will: on your own, or for someone else? **The fact is, you will never be RICH working for another.** However, you must crawl before you can walk.

Gym

All trainers have to cut their teeth, and a gym is a good place to do it. You get some really good experience with people and how the industry works as a whole. Working in the gym as a trainer was just a small part of a bigger plan. I sure learned a lot, mainly what NOT to do.

Learn the Ropes

I wanted to learn every aspect of the business, both from a trainer's point of view and an owner's. Over a period of time, here are the positions I worked:

Front Desk Attendant
Sales Coordinator
Marketing Coordinator
Floor Trainer
Fitness Director
Facility Controller
Janitor

Working in a gym is a necessary part of learning the fitness business, but there are some downsides and limitations to that, as well.

Self-Employed

My father was a farmer with a seventh-grade education. He never had a boss or owed a penny. We worked sixteen-hour days in the summer, but he taught us never to complain about any of it. If we did, he made us go work the summer for some one else. Ouch!

A few weeks ago, I sat across from the cutest couple at a restaurant. Not a care in the world, smiles on their faces and living life like tomorrow would ever come. I admired them so very much. My parents had worked hard all their lives, and it was their turn to enjoy it. What I admired most was the "FREEDOM" they enjoyed.

Trade-Offs

Working for others, they call the shots from scheduling to pay. I always felt no one had the right to do that. In the end, you have to decide: control or be controlled. I have been self-employed almost my entire life and pray that I always will be. But it comes with a price. Sure, it would have been emotionally easier for me to work for someone else and let them have all the stress, but I would have sacrificed much. The truth is, with FREEDOM and flexibility come longer hours and a tougher road. Sometimes you feel that you are on an island surrounded by sharks. Other times, the world is your oyster. There are no nine-to-five work hours; you eat, sleep and breathe your work.

-Self-Induced Stress

With having the freedom to call your own shots, also comes the stress of paying all the bills. You are responsible for everything. Even if you take one day off physically, mentally you are still there in the thick of it all. But it's yours and no one else's.

-Faith

Being self-employed requires faith, and at times a lot of it. You never know what each day will bring, good or bad. If you don't have faith in yourself, what you are doing and the path that's being taken, then you will not be successful. If you don't believe in yourself, no one else will, either.

-Guts

Self-employed people have guts; you must, too. Hard knocks make your spine stronger. Just as importantly, someone else would have controlled my income.

Freedom

The bottom line is, you must decide, *"What is the price you are willing to pay for having a little more freedom in life?"* I have a sign on my wall in front of my desk that reads:

Today I pray for:

> *Faith,*
> *Family,*
> *Freedom,*
> *Flexibility,*
> *Financial Peace,*
> *Fitness*

Today I am so very grateful and thankful for:

> *Faith,*
> *Family,*
> *Freedom,*
> *Flexibility,*
> *Financial Peace,*
> *Fitness*

Money Tips- Control everything, if possible—especially how much money you charge. Get experience in commercial settings, but in the end, the more freedom you have, the more money and happiness you will have.

45

My first million dollars was made with one treadmill, a row of DB, a stretching mat and a dream.

Greg Ryan

6
Profit- Size Does Matter

Yes, it's about Profit! As important as a business plan is, so is how I would treat success when it arrived. I was not doing this to fail, so I mapped out a plan beforehand. When success came, I did not spend much time on it. I developed a philosophy, *"Profit with Less."* For most trainers, it's not on the radar screen. If it's not, you will peter out.

Peter Principle 101

What does the phrase *"The Peter Principle"* mean? The term is used when an individual gets promoted into a position one level above what they are capable of handling. The Peter Principle can apply to either an individual or company. The health club and restaurant industry are notorious for the Peter Principle.

For whatever reason, usually arrogance and bad pride, an individual or company's short-term success has convinced them to have much larger aspirations. Unfortunately, such a mindset is usually the beginning of the end. Mismanagement, administrative errors or just too much responsibility to handle are all unforeseen mishaps. No one goes into business to fail, but growing too fast or getting too big to run effectively can sink the best of dreams in a hurry.

Work Smart, Not Hard

I treated my business like I treated my own fitness training: Work smart, not hard.

I became a successful bodybuilder very young, not because I was special or knew more, but because I worked more effectively in a much less amount of time than others.

Less Is More

If I could exercise smarter and get better results in half the time and effort, then why not have that same philosophy in business? To me, that's *common sense*. But I had to leave my pride and ego at the door no matter what opportunity came my way. This is not an easy thing to do when your business is thriving and you think, "Bigger business structure equals bigger bucks"—not so! Be very careful not to ride the wave of your ego!

My first million dollars was made with one treadmill, a row of DB, a stretching mat and a dream.

It's also worth noting that the *"Less is More"* attitude helped my average client retention to be eight years. My point is, don't make things complicated. Don't make things bigger for the sake of status, greed from ego.

There are three areas that are worth mentioning when having the attitude of less equals more: size of facility, equipment, and number of total clients you have.

Profit and Loss

Here is an example of the Peter Principle in the health club industry that happens all the time. Some gym owner makes some or a lot of money in a small facility (usually under ten thousand square feet), and they automatically build or rent a bigger one. They invest more time and money and hire additional employees, and very soon it's too much for them to handle.

They were better off staying relatively small and improving their profit margins.

Health clubs under ten thousand square feet traditionally make more money per square foot than those over ten thousand square feet.

Profit margin is the ratio of the cost of doing business to gross income. Sure, they may have grown the physical structure of their business or gym, but they are making less money overall and working twice as hard. In the end, they are only satisfying their ego all while their energy, love for the profession and personal life are being sucked dry. Not a good way to live.

You may think that this only applies to those owning or renting a facility — not so. You can see what's happening more clearly with them, but it can happen to the individual trainer, as well.

Profits by the Foot

From day one, I took the attitude:

"Try to make as much money with as little sweat, equity and overhead as I can."

My largest facility that I have owned consisted of two treadmills, one bike, an elliptical machine, a multi-weight stack machine and a row of dumbbells — three thousand square feet in total, believe it or not! Trainers have a hard time wrapping their heads around this one; that's why most are poor. If you get it, then you have a chance. My square footage profit is many times that of a gym of 50,000 square feet. That means more money in my pocket to do with as I please. Then I am a slave to no one.

Slave to the Lender

A great principle my father taught me was: *"You are a slave to the lender."* In other words, avoid bad debt at all costs. So, if you decide to have your own facility, here is the general rule: Rent the cardio, and buy the weight equipment. If you can buy all of it, do it, but many cannot swing that at first.

Remember two things: The less debt you have, the higher profits you have, and second, great customer service makes up for any lack of equipment or space.

Money Tip- Less is more! Square footage profit is more important than size. Bad debt is a burden to the business and soul; pay for as much as possible up front. Your ego will cost you thousands if you are not careful.

7
The Gatekeepers

Yes, it's about those around you! My father would say, *"You are only as good as those around you."* He always seemed to have good, quality friends and business associates around when he needed them.

Meet the Fockers — what a great movie. Jack (Robert De Niro) was always giving Greg (Ben Stiller) the business about <u>"The Circle of Trust."</u> Or in other words, a small family-like society of people who had your back no matter what. While earned, once in, you never would have to leave, unless you royally screwed up.

Your Circle of Trust

I always seemed to like team sports. Just watching a group of people come together for one common goal, fighting off adversity, or just playing for the love of the game was inspiring. It didn't matter as much about the outcome as it did what you learned about yourself and your teammates. You really are only as good at what you do as those you surround yourself with. You learned a lot about trust.

If you are going to run a profitable fitness business, you have to surround yourself with good, quality people; I call them my *"Gatekeepers."*

The Gatekeepers

These individuals possess better-than-average business knowledge and impeccable character. Gender, background or race matters not; it's about what's inside and upstairs.

The Mission

The goal of the so-called *Gatekeepers* is to help stay in line with the mission statement of your business. By the way, if you are serious about this *RICH TRAINER* thing, the first thing you should do is create a mission statement for your business. The second thing is to give you good sound business advice and then allow you to make a decision.

Quality, Not Quantity

The number of Gatekeepers is irrelevant; the type of people they are is more important. I have a diverse group that fits all of my business needs. You could have a few or many, as long as the goal is met.

-Trustworthy

Gatekeepers have to be trustworthy, of course. You need to count on them and not worry about things going on behind your back. Trust—not always an easy thing to read in people, is it?

-Loyal

Gatekeepers are loyal. You do not want someone on your side one day, and then flipping to someone else on another day. Loyalty also means not flip-flopping on principle. Everyone should believe in something, even if you don't agree on it.

-Bold

Gatekeepers need a spine. They must be bold in their beliefs and convictions, and committed to the cause.

-Straight Shooters

I don't like fluff; just give it to me straight. Gatekeepers have to be straight shooters and tell it like it is.

The Key Holders

I had a game plan of who I wanted guarding my business gates. I only wanted a selected few key holders that consisted of people who specialized in important areas of my business.

Mentor

A mentor is a coach, counselor or teacher whom you respect and look up to for advice. In a perfect world, they should be one in your profession. If you can meet on a consistent basis with a person you consider a mentor, that will be priceless. Kathy Smith, the famous fitness guru, was my mentor.

Accountability Partner

An accountability partner (AP) is a person who holds you to your goals and mission of your company. You meet on a regular basis, more so than a mentor. An AP is not a mentor, and a mentor is not an AP. Whether you know it or not, you get off track at times and need a friendly GPS to get you back on track, and like it or not, an AP can and should do that.

CPA

This goes without saying, but you need a trustworthy CPA.

Financial Planner

A financial planner is different than a CPA. A financial planner helps you with strategic planning of finances in the future. It should go along with your mission statement of your company. If you are serious about your future, then why not have a gatekeeper who helps you plan ahead on your finances, as well?

No Family Members

A good rule of thumb is: Do NOT have family members as gatekeepers. Family and business in ninety-five percent of the time do not mix. What starts out as good intentions ends in wedges splitting the best of families apart, sometimes for good.

Whoever the people are guarding your gates, remember that it's about quality, not quantity. **Gatekeepers can be the difference between freedom and poverty.**

Money Tip- You are only as good as those around you. Protect your interests with wise counsel. Money not spent is money earned. Realize that you cannot do it all alone. Learn from those before you, and always cover your butt.

8
The Law of the Few

Yes, less is more! Some people call it the eighty-twenty rule. I like the way Malcolm Gladwell explains it in his book *The Tipping Point*. He calls it *"The Law of the Few."*

With the Oprah Winfrey attitude of structuring an empire and my father's gatekeeper mentality of protecting the fort, I developed my own business template or philosophy to fit the fitness business. **In the long term, I wanted to create a system that I could duplicate anywhere at any time.**

A Business Template

A *"Business Template"* is a certain way you choose to conduct your business—a mold, manual or guide, so to speak. My philosophy has always been simple:

Work smart and develop quality relationships with people, organizations and companies, spending as little on advertising as possible.

In other words, create a group or network around you that works with and for your business 24/7. A *Network* is any netlike system that connects things, objects or people together. The Oprah approach and the gatekeepers are only as good for your business as the quality of people they allow *through*.

The Law of the Few

Growing up on a farm, we sold our produce to a local market that distributed fruit and vegetables all over the country. In the beginning, we had to go to the market to sell our crops.

Over time, my father developed meaningful relationships with selected buyers there. He knew the importance of cultivating and nurturing not only his crops, but relationships, as well. I just didn't seem to have his personality. Interestingly enough, I noticed that he only spent time with a selected few; they were sought out every time we went there. At the time, I never understood why. Now I do!

During harvesting time, we would get consistent calls from the *selected few* buyers, each one placing substantial orders for our produce. As long as I can remember, those few individuals supplied us with all the orders we could handle without leaving our farm. Those few made my father a ton of cash. Malcolm Gladwell explains it in *The Law of the Few* like this:

"The majority of the work will be done by a handful of exceptional people who have the appropriate skill sets."

He goes onto say that there are three key types of people in the majority—connectors, mavens, and salesman—each having a different role to play.

The main goal was to find a **"few"** quality people, organizations or companies to send me clients, and have them come to me when at all possible. If a connector (one who was good at *networking),* a maven (an up-to-date *information* geek) and a salesman (someone good at *persuasion*) happened to be in the fold, then that was icing on the cake.

Observing my father convinced me that if you only even had a few good ones, they could and would supply you with as much business as you would ever need. Looking back, my father also taught me the smart way to fish.

Fish for the Big Ones

When fishing for the big ones, you first spend time finding a great hole to fish out of. When you find it, stay there until you feel you've caught all the keepers. In other words, ask yourself:

"Who and what organizations, companies and professions have the same or similar customer, client or patient base that I want?"

What professions are the fertile ponds, and who in those professions are the biggest fish? Here are the professions (ponds) I caught the biggest fish out of:

Orthopedic Surgeons
Physical Therapist/Occupational Therapist
Psychologist
Nutritionists
Endocrinologist
Spas

Fitness trainers make the mistake of going back to the same pond or gym thinking that clients are just going to appear. The gym has been all fished out. So, the first part of a good fitness training business template is to build a group of quality like-minded professionals that you can network with. **This group, if nurtured and developed, can and will send you all the clients you will need, and guess what? For FREE.**

A word of caution: Make sure that they share the same philosophy and similar goals for their clients/customers you do. This is very important for your long-term success.

Create a Win-Win

The best posturing you can have when you approach someone is to create a win-win relationship. Without making it noticeable, emphasize what you and your business can and will do to enhance their patients, customers, organizations or institutions.

Home Field Advantage

In any negotiating or sports event for that matter, you will have an advantage if it's on your own turf—you know the terrain. The second part of developing your template is to get them to come to you. This has many unseen benefits to you and your company, from scheduling, perceived value, comfort, confidence and retention. This is one area where having your own facility is a big plus.

Referral Base Business

When people tell you that referrals are the cheapest way of getting new people through your door, they're not kidding. This type of business template has saved me more time, effort and money over the years than I can put a figure to. Nurture the relationships, and the rest will follow. Practicing the "Law of a Few" was one of the best things I have ever done in my business.

Money Tip- Spend less on outside advertisement by having a few good referral base people around you. A small number of good like-minded people can send you all the business you will ever need.

9
Bottoms Up

Yes, you must have structure! With anything, if there is no firm foundation, then everything will perish sooner or later. If you are sold out and truly respect what you are planning on accomplishing, you must from the beginning have structure, both personally and professionally. Legal, administrative, policies, and pricing are all important and vital parts to a successful, fully functioning fitness business.

I cannot overestimate the importance of implementing and following through with the day-to-day structure of your business. *Having the greatest, sold out attitude without business structure is meaningless. And without such an attitude, your structure will not grow.*

Legal Framework

Setting up your business from a legal standpoint will vary from state to state, but here are some basics to think about.

Limited Liability Corporation- LLC

Right from the beginning, I set up a LLC or Limited Liability Corporation, and I'm glad that I did. I gained more respect for what I was doing and helped cover my butt if anything bad happened in my facilities or to another person.

Insurance

It is a good common practice to acquire some sort of accidental liability insurance.

Usually a millions dollars of coverage is enough, but that will vary from business to business.

Employees

I always preferred to subcontract all my employees out; there are tax advantages in doing so, among other benefits. Unless your business gets to a certain size, part-time subcontractors are best.

Money Tip- CYA! Make sure that you have legal coverage in preparation of any situation or circumstances.

10
Principle Makes Policy

Yes, it's about principles. You can have the best attitude, philosophy, legal structure, and facility (if you chose), but without sound day-to-day business policies and procedures, success will not be in the cards for you.

Policies

This is an area that may vary. Each trainer, owner, or director may have different ways of doing and implementing policies, and that's fine. As we keep the bigger picture in mind, let me share with you a few things that have worked for me: consistency and simplicity.

Simplicity

Whatever policies you develop in your training business, be sure that they are simple to implement. More importantly, make it easy for your customers and clients to follow. *This will save you energy and effort, and will increase your client retention in the end.*

Consistency

No matter what policies you draw up, make sure that you are consistent in implementing them. You will be tested in every single way possible. If you are inconsistent with enforcing them, you will immediately lose credibility—not only from your clients, but within yourself, as well.

Hours of Operation

This one varies for everyone, as well. I always had a set time when I made appointments, and each potential client was educated as to the times when I was open for business. Over the years, I learned not to take phone calls past a certain hour. If you are in business for yourself, you realize that you are always thinking about the business; however, you have to learn how to manage your thinking, as well.

My personal life was my business, and my professional life was at selected times during the day and maybe weekends. Whatever you decide, stick with it, even when you are tested and/or need the money.

Scheduling

One thing I learned early on was: Control your schedule.

When a client wanted to make an appointment, I asked them, *"When do you want to come in?"* instead of giving them two options on my terms. I guess I was afraid that they wouldn't like my times. Then I realized that they respected me more if I took charge, and I felt better about time management.

Cancellation and No-shows

Some trainers think that I'm harsh on my cancellation and no-show policy, but guess what? It works, and works big-time. I enforce a twenty-four hour cancellation policy, period. They are handed a policy sheet at the first orientation, and it is followed from that moment forward. If they do not cancel, they are charged; by the way, they all pay up front, as well. The only exception to this rule is in the case of sickness.

And they damn well better actually be sick if they're going to claim sickness. By implementing such a policy, I have almost no cancellations and no second-guessing in my weekly schedule.

No-shows

I have not had one for as long as I can remember. Why is that? I treat my business like a business. The client sees that, so they take it more seriously.

Three Strikes, You're Out

I some cases, I have to enforce a business rule that I don't like, the *"Three Strikes, You're Out"* policy. While difficult, it must be done for my mental health and for the business. Failing to show or canceling three times in the same time period shows me that they don't care like they should.

I am not in business to take a people's money or to babysit an adult. This may sound harsh, but it keeps me in control of my business, and I don't enable them by allowing them to disrespect my time and theirs.

Dress Codes

Some of this may sound over the top, but I realized a few things about what people would wear that affected their workouts and how long they stayed with me. While to most trainers, it would not matter nor would they even have a clue as to what was really going on, it translated into dollars, I discovered.

Mostly I don't care what people wear; if it's comfortable to them, then fine. But, being too comfortable ended up getting in the way. There are only two things that I will not allow for clients to wear while working out: jeans and open-toed shoes. I have two reasons for not allowing jeans: limited movement, and lack of respect or seriousness in regard to their session. Limited movement most can understand, but the latter, lack of respect—What the heck does that mean? I learned over the years that wearing jeans was a sure sign that the client was going to quit working out with me in the near future.

They had lost interest and were now not making it a priority. First, it's the shoes—I can handle that once in a while—but when they would start to wear jeans, then I knew that they were on a slippery slope and soon would stop working out with me. So, I did not allow it, period.

The only exception to the rules was their age. If they are over sixty-five, then fine. Maybe a little inconsistent with policy, but elderly people usually don't quit; they just want to be comfortable and not inconvenienced by changing clothes twice a day. I don't blame them, in a way. Now, opened-toed shoes are just a safety thing. If they or I dropped a weight on their foot, ouch! And that could, in the end, be a liability. I am flexible in most things, but with those two I'm not.

Cell Phones

Now, here is a touchy one. We live in an instant information world. Everyone wants to or thinks they have to stay in touch with everything and everyone.

I have news for them: They don't. I explain my reasons right up front as to why I do NOT allow cell phones while working out. They can place it in another room within hearing distance, but cannot carry it on their persons. There are cases of emergency—I understand that—but most of the time, they are just a pain. I try to explain that it's a good time for quiet time for them.

Money Tips- Any business needs structure. Guidelines and policies are frameworks for less cash left on the table and more energy to build wealth.

Your income is in relationship to your self-worth!

11
Pricing for Profit

Yes, it's about money! I want to speak on this topic in its own chapter because I feel it's important enough to do so. There are many things that go into pricing a fitness trainer service. Most of the time, trainers will leave a lot of money on the table; I sure have over the years.

No Used Car Salesman

Do not shop prices out. In other words, they are what they are. Make a decision, and stick to it. Do not change or give one person a certain price and the other a different one. If you do, it cheapens your service, you don't feel good about yourself, and bet your boots other clients will find out if you undercut them or not.

No Negotiating

In this business, there is no negotiating. There is no reason to negotiate; your prices are what they are. The art of it all is a negotiating principle: Tell your price, and then shut up!! He who speaks first, loses. I talked too much and ended up apologizing in so many words for my price, in the end leaving money on the table. They would have paid my first price, but I assumed that they would or could not.

DO NOT ASSUME THAT THEY CANNOT AFFORD YOU. If they don't buy from you, it's a timing thing, not an affordability issue.

Those same people will walk out your door and into a car dealership and plop down thousands for a car.

No Horse Trading

I see personal trainers do this a lot: They *"Horse Trade."* In other words, they swap out things for services. Some people call it bartering. I call it "Not Smart!"

On the surface, bartering seems like a win-win proposition. You get something of value you want or need, and the other party gets your time. Almost seems like you are getting something you want for free, doesn't it? Well, you're not. You are paying a price, and you don't even realize it.

In the end, you discount the value or your service, you don't feel good about yourself, they tell others you are a freebie, and you have to manage your schedule; they no-show a lot. No matter how much you want or need their product, don't horse trade. I haven't bartered in thirty years, not once.

No "Pay as You Go"

Mostly, I have always had a policy of getting people to pay up front. In the beginning of my career, I was just thankful to have any type of client, so I was lenient on my payment plan. Once again, I left a lot of money on the table. I also found that "pay as you go" clients canceled more often.

No Credit, No Service

This one is a tough one. It really comes down to your philosophy about your business.

On the one hand, I could make more money by clients charging on their credit cards. I found that there are more cancelations and no-shows. Charging fitness training sessions on credit cards is like health insurance policies. When you go for the service, you feel like it's free because it's not necessarily directly out of your pocket. In other words, when people paid for sessions by credit card, they would not take it very seriously; there was no pain from the pocket.

On the front end, it looks like you are making more dough, but in the end you have to collect, track sessions, and manage no-shows and cancellations. It's not worth the hassle.

Perceived Value

There is a psychology to pricing your services. Have you ever said to yourself after learning what someone makes, *"How in the world would someone pay that person that much for that job? He's not worth that!"* Well, he thinks that he is, and that's all that matters.

KNOW THIS!

When I first moved to Los Angeles, I found out pretty quickly what a lack of self-worth had cost me for the last four years as a fitness trainer. I landed a dream job with fitness guru Kathy Smith's health club in Santa Monica, California. Working there for a month with about twenty other trainers—some not qualified, others good talkers, and a few knew their stuff—I asked one of the more successful ones to lunch.

I wanted to know what I needed to do to. They passed the looks test, there wasn't anything special about them, yet they were making hundreds of dollars an hour. How?

After chatting a while, Steven said to me, *"Double your price."* What? Double my price! Yes, he said firmly. That sent chills up my spine. *"Understand, I am a small-town boy just thankful to get paid something for exercising with people."* I said.

Steven says, *"It's about perceived value."* Whether you are worth what you are asking or not is really not a decision of yours; it's the potential client's. If you charge more, they think you are more knowledgeable and better from their point of view. If the market can bear your price, then people will pay for it. The very thought of doubling my session price was frightening. I was having a hard time as it was; now I really was going to run people off, so I thought. But, I wanted what he had. I didn't much respect his training tactics, but I did see his client list. So, I doubled my price.

In less than a month and a half, I had doubled my client load and income at the same time. Unbelievable! Needless to say, I got over that fear pretty quickly. I learned about two things: perceived value, and better customer service.

Better Service

I understood Steven's points of perceived value, but what we didn't discuss is what happened later. As I charged more, I felt that I had better give more to the customer than what they expected, so I did. Then when I raised my prices again, they had absolutely no problem with it. And the cycle continued: better service, higher income. Two very valuable lessons on pricing were learned in 1991: **Charge what you think you are worth — no more, no less — and your service should always exceed your pricing.**

Money Tip – Don't be a used car salesman. Stick with a pricing program no matter what. No freebies up front, only on the back end of an agreement. Charge what you think you are worth, period.

Never take for granted OJT, and never neglect Ph.D.

12
Education (Ph.D.) vs. Motivation (OJT)

Yes, it's about getting educated! The fitness industry hosts a wide range of characters. In general, the profession does not fully require institutional degrees, but does encourage some form of certification or formal education. The industry has left such requirements up to each organization, company or individual. So the debate, Ph.D. or OJT, goes on.

More Options, More Money

For what its worth, my opinion is that you *should* have some form of organized sponsored education. It helps build a stronger foundation to your business and could open up opportunities you may never had otherwise. As you learned with the Oprah approach, the more options you have at your fingertips, the more income streams you can create.

Being in business for myself most of my career, I can honestly say in thirty years I might have been asked about my classroom education fewer than two dozen times. On the other hand, having it helped me open up at least a dozen doors that I can think of off the top of my head.

Education (Ph.D.)

The college institutional system has yet to totally buy into some form of degreed fitness training program. Over the past ten years, there have, however, been a number of sponsored accredited programs that have risen in popularity.

Some hold more weight in the community than others, but in the end, it's up to you to which you chose to pursue.

American College of Sports Medicine

If status and prestige are your thing, then the program of certification you want is from the America College of Sports Medicine, or A.C.S.M. This certification is looked upon by those in the industry as the be-all and end-all of certifications. The thing is, it's a very challenging program, and most people opt for a lower-level educational program due to the industry's lack of requirements.

ACE

Another program is the American College of Exercise. If the A.C.S.M. is not your interest, this one may be your next choice — a very reputable program.

NFPT

The last one I will mention is the National Federation of Personal Trainers. This is another popular certification program worth looking into.

Paperweights

A word of caution about the rest of the programs marketed out there. While educational programs are worth completing, be sure to do homework first on which one is best for you.

Motivation (OJT)

I am a big advocate of getting a classroom education to increase your options and knowledge, but there is much more to being successful as a trainer. Like I have stated, this book is worth a million dollars to me because of what I have learned in the trenches over the past thirty years. There is no better teacher than OJT, or *"On-the-Job Training."*

To be in the RICH TRAINER category, one must possess both education and experience, and this may just take some time.

Money Tips- More options means more opportunity to make money. But does it mean that more degrees equals more money? That's debatable. Get your degree or certification, and move on. Do not hide behind them, or you will not make money.

On-the-job training is priceless; it's the real world. Combine classroom education and real-world experience, and the money will follow.

By the way, if you are serious about this RICH TRAINER thing, the first thing you should do is create a mission statement for your business.

Business 101 Review

Making money as a trainer comes down to attitude. Don't be a sellout; be "Sold Out" to your profession, while at the same time acting as a professional. In most cases, try to control your destiny, and structure and run your business with boundaries supported by good, sound business principles.

Protect your interests with Gatekeepers and Mentors while avoiding a used car salesman reputation. In the end, it's your on-the-job training that will teach you more than a book, but never neglect a good institutional education. Becoming wealthy as fitness trainer is a mind thing; treat it as such in every way. Fitness training is a business; treat it as such in every way. Never take for granted OJT, and never neglect Ph.D.

Attitude- Lifer or nothing.
Theme- It's a profession; treat it as such.
Tagline- The "Foundation" of Wealth

Sell Out or be Sold Out — You pick it!

III

Trainer Ethics 101

The "Right" Stuff for Success

Trainer Ethics 101 Overview

How you conduct your fitness training career is your business. But, understand that life will have its say sooner or later. The success of the business is up to you, not your clients; *how you go about getting it may be more important than the wealth, status or experience that you want to acquire.*

Ethics, by definition, are moral principles you have inside you. Your actions, at their core, are determined by such morals, and life will either reward you for them or turn on you because of them. Your ethical beliefs affect yourself, others and your profession as a whole—remember that. Each day you will have to decide; follow what is right, even when it may not be popular, or compromise everything for the sake of the moment or circumstances. We live and die by our daily decisions.

13
The "Right" Thing

Yes, it's about doing the *"Right"* thing. How you conduct your fitness training career is your business, but understand that life will have its say, sooner or later. The success of your business is up to you, not your clients; how you go about getting it may be more important than the wealth, status or experience that you want to acquire.

Do the "Right" Thing

Ethics, by definition, are moral principles you have inside you. Your actions, at their core, are determined by such morals. Life will either reward you for them or turn on you because of them. Your ethical beliefs affect you, others and your profession as a whole—remember that. Each day you will have to decide: *"Follow what is right in your heart, even if unpopular, or compromise everything for the sake of the moment or circumstances."*

I have tried my best to let actions speak for my mouth; this has not always been easy. I've learned that actions are the best form of leadership for people and clients. Make sure that your actions align with your belief system, too.

Permission to Say No

A lot of trainers don't want to appear weak by not knowing an answer to a question. The right thing to do is tell them that you don't know, but you will find the answer out for them. Respecting them and yourself is better in the long run. **Dishonesty only brings strife and poverty to your heart and business.**

No Hypocrites

Doing the right thing sometimes means doing what is unpopular. Don't just say one thing and do another just to appease people.

Political Correctness

Political correctness in the fitness business is an enabler. Whatever you believe, stand up for it. Don't be a wishy-washy trainer. Your clients and other people may not agree with you, but they will respect you and your opinion.

What Goes Around Comes Around

The truth about Karma is that it's real. Do not undercut, backstab or talk about another trainer or fitness profession; it will only make you and the profession look and feel bad.

14
Actions Speak Volumes

Yes, it's about actions. Ethics-*the moral principles of an individual.* In other words, *do the RIGHT thing, even when it is not popular.* Following this type of attitude is one of the hardest things to do, day in and day out.

Having good, sound principles in your business is just as important for you personally as it is for the reputation of your business. Your business is an extension of you. If you are ethical in your personal life, you will be on the up-and-up in your business life. Sooner or later, unethical pursuits of success will crush your world.

A Right Thing Gone Wrong

In the spring of 1988, I won my last bodybuilding contest; that summer, I retired at the top of my game, but at a low point in my ethical life. In the fall of that same year, I went public with my addiction to anabolic steroids. Right or wrong, I felt like a hypocrite. Sure, it's part of the fabric of competitive sports as a whole, but it doesn't justify my personal decision to take illegal drugs.

I was not doing the right thing, and it had been eating at me for months. My goal in bodybuilding from the beginning was to build my self-esteem and confidence more so than my biceps or thighs; honestly it was. So, retiring at the top of my game was not hard. For most, knowing when to stop haunts them for their entire career. But somewhere along the way, what started out with the right intentions went wrong.

Stopping the drug use was the *right* thing to do. Unfortunately, it took me two more years to follow through on my promise to myself; my cousin's dying of a steroid-related cancer may have had something to do with that.

Not a Popularity Contest

There are times in life when you should do the right thing even if it's not politically correct with society, peers or even closer family members. At the end of the day, you have to live with yourself, and the opinion of others is just that: Everyone has one.

Practice True Character

True character comes when you do the "right" thing when no one is watching.

A trainer called me up yesterday and wanted to rent out one of my training studios. I asked if they were working for another trainer in town, and she said yes. I mentioned that I was fully open to the idea, but I needed to speak with the trainer she was working with first, out of courtesy. She didn't quite understand that. So, needless to say, she never rented from me. No ethics, no business!

15
Profession Courtesy

Yes, it's about courtesy! We spoke about this earlier and the importance of loving and respecting what you do, but it goes much deeper. *Over time, a majority of fitness trainers have cast a bad light on the profession itself.*

Professional- *of, relating to, or characteristic of a profession, engaged in one of the learned professions, characterized by or conforming to the technical or ethical standards of a profession*

Bad Apples

Let's say you have a bad experience with a particular service, such as a carpet cleaning. The next time you need your carpets cleaned, what will be the first thing you think of? Getting bad service again! You can't help but have a bad taste in your mouth about the entire industry because of your experience; right or wrong, you lose confidence and even respect for that person, business or profession.

Acting like a *professional* really means doing what it takes to make others think of you as reliable, respectful, and competent. Acting like a professional covers everything we have talked about so far. Acting like a professional has common traits.

Competence- You're good at what you do, and you have the skills and knowledge that enable you to do your job well.

Reliability- People can depend on you to show up on time, submit your work when it's supposed to be ready, etc.

Honesty- You tell the truth and are up-front about where things stand.

Integrity- You are known for your consistent principles.

Respect for Others- Treating all people as if they mattered is part of your approach.

Supporting Others- You share the spotlight with colleagues, take time to show others how to do things properly, and lend an ear when necessary.

I cannot express to you the importance of respecting your profession by acting like a professional. Your actions will mean far more than you will ever know. Do us all a favor: If you are not willing to treat the fitness training profession with respect, get out now. Please! And especially do not become one of these......

16
Beware the Wolf Spider

Yes, it's about competing within yourself! Why do so many trainers in the profession act like they are threatened or something? Other trainers are not your enemy. You are the biggest threat to your business. So, why do you feel threatened?

The "Wolf Spider" Syndrome

Have you ever heard of a wolf spider? Have you ever seen a wolf spider? Most never have. Why? They are few in numbers and small in stature, all for a reason. Wolf spiders are one of the only species that *"Eat their own."* They are ruthless, selfish, moment-to-moment thinkers, insecure, prideful, paranoid small-town creatures.

They have no sense of the big picture whatsoever. Without calling out specific professions, there are a lot of people in the medical and fitness industry that resemble a Wolf Spider. People with wolf spider behaviors spend most of their energy in the competitive side of life rather than the creative side. Let me say it again,

"If you have one or many Wolf Spider tendencies, you will stay broke, unhappy, and in the end, full of resentment. Is this what you really want to become?"

You have got to get a hold of your mind and manage it.

Managing the ID/EGO

There is nothing wrong with *taking* pride in something; that means that you care. On the flip side, bad pride comes from your EGO or ID. Singlehandedly, your EGO can break your career; maybe not all of a sudden or even noticeably, but getting above your business will sink you—I promise you that.

Be grateful and humble, and for God's sake stop thinking that you know it all. Besides, people know when you are giving them a line of crap.

You can easily complicate your path to wealth by driving out common sense with too much other stuff, especially pride and EGO. Be very, very careful not to leave thousands on the table by trying to be a know-it-all!

Trainer Ethics 101 Review

You are only as good you are when no one is watching. Do the *"Right"* thing in your heart first. Practice being different rather than the norm; it makes more money, anyway. Take pride in being an expert, and be professional at all costs. In the end, you will pay dearly if you don't.

Let your actions speak so loudly that when you do eventually say something, they cannot hear you. And whatever you do, don't become the Wolf Spider and eat your own.

Attitude- You get what you give.
Theme- Do the right thing, even when not popular.
Tagline- The "Right" Thing for Success

Strangle the competitive, and Nurture the Creative!

IV
Psychology 101

The "Creative" Process to Prosperity in Fitness

Psychology 101 Overview

Not only is psychology a part of the success of your clients, it is a vital part of the process with in yourself—maybe even more so. Competition comes not from the world as much as it does from you.

Despite what you might think or have been taught, you attract success or poverty based on what you believe to be true or not. Free your mind, and the rest will follow. Nurture the creative and imaginative, and success cannot help but cross your path. The best way to do this is by looking outward and helping others, and at the same time looking inward to help yourself.

Like I said in the beginning, becoming wealth as a fitness trainer is more about your mind than the next great workout program.

17
Free Your Mind

Yes, wealth is created in the mind first! *It's not about you,* when it comes to the success of your <u>clients.</u> *It IS all about you* when it comes to the success of your <u>business.</u>

"Yes, it's a business, and yes, it's personal."

Let's face it: You are the business, and the product or service is provided by you. Maybe one of the most challenging things ever to sell is HOPE, FAITH and MOTIVATION. Selling the invisible is more of a mental negotiation between you and the person you are speaking with. You must first sell or believe it yourself.

In the end, it's not about you; it's about taking care of the client. However, in the very beginning, even before you meet a potential client, it starts with you and your thinking.

The secret to wealth as a fitness trainer comes from within. Making money comes from the mind. There are many financial gurus and Fortune 500 CEOs who believe that creating wealth is eighty percent mental and twenty percent action. Building a nice nest egg is more about HOW you feel about money than anything. If you think that the green stuff is a good, more will enter into your life. If you feel that it's the root of all evil, you will continue to lack it.

Small-town Thinking

Growing up in a small town hindered the financial part of my business for a short period of time. A smaller environment doesn't necessarily lend itself to bigger dreams for the most part.

A majority of people become prisoners in their own minds. It's no fault of their own; it's a learned way of thinking that they have no other options. Something learned, however, can be unlearned.

Too Close to Home

Remember my story about pricing and perceived value, that stemmed from my small-town thinking? It was a really hard lesson learned. Sometimes it takes looking at situations from the outside to become aware of what is really going on inside. I happened to be too close to home, so to speak, to realize how much my small-town thinking was affecting my personal, professional and financial growth.

The best thing that happened for my career was moving to California. I did not realize it at that moment, but getting away from what I had become accustomed to helped me to become aware of what was mentally hindering my business. **Financial prosperity in the fitness business is directly linked to how you view the world, imagination/creativity, and your belief in who you are and what you do.**

I will talk about this more in length later, but it is worth briefly mentioning here in this chapter:

Learning the X's and O's on an exercise chart or how to monitor heart rates is only about twenty percent of what makes a successful trainer. The other eighty percent is mental.

FREE YOUR MIND, AND THE REST WILL FOLLOW!

18
Competitive to Creative

Yes, wealth is about being creative, not competitive! On a personal note, a while back I was diagnosed with ADHD or Attention Deficit Hyperactive Disorder, a neurological issue with the brain. I liken it to an idling high-revving engine. For years my brain was in overdrive, always ten steps ahead of my body. One of many things I learned, I believe, is appropriate to what it takes to be a successful and even wealthy trainer.

In order for me to manage my ADHD with or without the aid of medication, I had to learn to utilize one part of my brain more than another. The more I was in the right side or creative side, the better I would function, enjoy life and attract better things into it. I had to be more imaginative, in other words.

I learned that one of the main things that exacerbated my ADHD was left-brain thinking, overanalyzing even a competitive mindset. More importantly, I realized that my thinking, ADHD or not, was working against me. Moving forward, I had to find a daily mental exercise to get me from the competitive, self-centered side of my head to the creative and imaginative side — the freer one. As weird as this may sound, even though I had become successful as a trainer, I did it the hard way mentally.

I believe that this chapter is the most important one of this whole book!

Your success is not about what you do, but how you think.

Competitive Thinking

A host of a nationally syndicated radio station asked me yesterday, "What two things hinder a trainer from being successful?" Without hesitation I said, **"Ego and small-town thinking!"** In other words: *"Competitive Thinking."*

This will be one of the hardest daily challenges you will ever try to master. I said, "try," because most will not even try, or will give up after a few days or will consider it weird and pointless. Let me tell you, your biggest competitor is not others; it's yourself. The only one you should be concerned with is you. *"Competitive Thinking" is when you spend most of your time worrying about what others are doing, and not on what you can do better. Competitive thinking is spending too much time in your left brain.*

There is nothing wrong with logic and reason, but too much of it and not enough imagination or creativity dulls the mind and hinders your success as a trainer — believe me when I say that.

Creative Thinking

Creative thinking comes from the right side of the brain. It's more free-spirited, imaginative and inspirational. From a psychological standpoint, you cannot become successful without utilizing your creative, imaginative side.

It's Not about Numbers

Learning the X's and O's on an exercise chart and how to monitor heart rates is only about twenty percent of what makes a successful trainer. The rest is psychology. Yes, calories in and calories out play a large role in contributing to people's fitness levels, there is no denying that.

However, if you get too hung up on the charts (left brain) you will lose clients.

Both Points of View

There are two points of view that are very important when it comes to being a RICH trainer: dealing with your mindset and the client's mindset. Learning how the psychology of how you tick and how the clients tick is vital to your success. The most important thing is learning how YOU think.

You must, I say it again, **"You must learn how to not be competitive with yourself, others and the world in general. Competitive thinking only hinders greatness coming into your life. Creativity and imagination spring forth opportunities daily."**

"When the student is ready, the teacher appears," I once read.

You don't have, because you don't ask. Why is that?

Greg Ryan

19
The Law of Attraction

I don't usually promote books within my own books, but I want to share with you a mindset that over the years has changed my life, business, and the way I see life as a whole.

In the bestselling book *The Secret*, Rhonda Bryne explains how we basically attract things into our lives by our thoughts, persona and behaviors. We don't intentionally wish for bad or good things to come into our lives, but if we step back and listen to our speech, see our actions and feel our feelings, we would be shocked at all of them. It would help us to understand the events and circumstances of our past.

I personally believe that we are our biggest competitor, more in our mind than anything. I also have come to think that whether we understand it or not, we attract the good and bad into our lives. The only thing keeping you from being a successful and even wealthy trainer is your thinking. Whatever we think, we get. Sounds simple, doesn't it?

I want you to take a moment and step outside of yourself and circumstances. Focus on your conversations not only with people, but in your head.

Becoming a successful trainer is more about what's in your head than on the charts!

The Attractive Process

In the previous chapter, we learned about the power of creativity verses the hindrance of competitive thinking. If you want to attract people, things or business into your life, you have to get and stay in the creative side. You have to come up with mind games by using your imagination on a daily basis. Here are some key areas in bringing business and prosperity into your life:

Ask

People in general, and trainers especially, are afraid to ask for help or clients. You don't *have* because you don't *ask*, someone once said. Swallow the pride and ask your Creator, the world and individuals for exactly what you want.

Believe/Have Faith

I know some of this stuff you've heard, but it is so much of a part of being successful in anything in life. There may be no other profession in life requiring some sort of belief and faith that you are doing the right thing.

Let's face it: You are selling hope, and your potential customers, by their very nature, do not want to exercise. You really, truly have to believe in yourself and what you are doing, and know that prosperity is coming. Every day, you have to have very strong faith in the unseen. I could tell you story after story of times when my belief system was empty, yet out of the blue it became apparent that people, things and income potentials were going on behind the scenes to better me and my business.

Visualization

I am convinced that your mind's eye is one of the most powerful tools in attracting things into your world. I have gone so far as writing myself fake checks as visualization techniques to boost my imagination; I then pasted them on my office wall so to look at them daily. Numerous times I have received that same about from a client not too long after that. Say what you will, but it works. I fully accredit my bodybuilding success to this technique. I could share stories on how visualization changed my physical body right before my very eyes.

Intentions

People have good or bad intentions in doing things. If you ask for something of this world, make sure that you have good intentions behind it. Bad intentions usually don't bring about a prosperous life.

-Intend It

There is something to be said about the power of the "will." Not willpower, but how you will things into existence.

This NCAA basketball tournament is going on right now. It is amazing to watch some teams just will themselves into winning. The mindset can apply to your fitness training prosperity, as well. There is a lot of pull in getting what you want, if you will or intend it into your life.

There is a so-called chassis that runs most things. You can believe, have faith, use your imagination and will until you are blue in the face, but there is one thing that is the key to attracting prosperity into your life and business.

Gratitude

No matter where you are in life, what you have or don't have, you must be grateful. Gratitude is the key to prosperity.

My career has had its ups and downs. It's certainly a lot easier to be grateful in the good times than in the bad times. But no matter the circumstances, you have to find a way to show gratitude. Good things will not come to you unless you are grateful for what you already have.

The first thing I do each morning is list off the things I am grateful for. If a bad mood exists or anxiety about my business is in the air, focusing on gratitude pretty much immediately changes the paradigm of my mind, allowing creativity to flow and attract new ideas, people and money.

The Secret in a Nutshell

The bottom line is that you don't get everything in life you deserve, but everything in life everything you *attract*. Seriously, if you stepped foot outside yourself and listened to how you talk and even knew how you think on a daily basis, it would make you sick. You may not want to admit it, but you do attract everything in your life.

Remember my story about doubling my price in L.A.? When I first moved there, I was attracting twenty-dollar-an-hour clients; that was just my mentality. I did not believe that I was worth more, so that's what the world gave me. You might not understand this (and you obviously don't or else you would be writing your own books), but **you have to be a millionaire in your head before you are one on paper!**

I never in my wildest dreams thought that someone would just write me a check for thousands of dollars. Today, it's the norm. And I love it!

Money Tip: Your success is not determined by what others think you are worth. Making money is about what *you* think you deserve and are worth, and how you attract it into your life.

Psychology 101 Review

Building wealth is mental more than physical. In order to accomplish that, you must first teach your brain how to think differently than most, as well as differently from what you are accustom to. Your enemy or competitor is none other than you. The more you can be creative and less concerned about others, the better.

Whether you believe it or not and even think it's weird, it's true; you attract good, bad, money or poverty into your life. We play a dangerous game by the way we think. I can attest, visualizing works! If you want to build wealth, you have to believe it and see it first. The main chassis that runs your mind and money is *"Gratitude."*

Attitude- Free your mind and the rest will follow.
Theme- Acquiring cash is mental more than physical.
Tagline- The Creative Process to Prosperity.

V

Common Sense 101

The "Approach" to Making Real Money

Common Sense 101 Overview

Ignorance is the absence of common sense. Unfortunately, common sense is not learned; you either possess it, or you don't. To be a success in fitness training, practicing good judgment is as important as exercising is to losing weight.

Fitness training is a people business, and that requires common-sense approaches. Without it you will fail, not because of your effort, but due to a disconnection between you and the client. Incorporate a little dose of common sense into your teaching methods, and you will be shocked at how easy your profession can become.

20
The Price of Ignorance

Yes, having common sense is priceless! *Ignorance is the absence of common sense!* In the real world, all the education will not make you successful unless you have a little common sense in your approach to being a fitness trainer. This is such a problem with fitness trainers that I felt it warranted a chapter of its own.

Practice Good Judgment

Common sense, by definition, means *sound and prudent judgment based on a simple perception of the situation or facts.* Common sense is where someone's fantasy world meets the real world. So, what causes a lack of common sense?

Fitness trainers spend so much energy focusing on the classroom and the scientific side of things that they miss the emotional real-life areas that will make them more successful in the end. Unfortunately, I believe that common sense cannot be taught; you either have the ability to communicate on a level of understanding or you don't. **Your success may just come down to how well you can encourage and hold people accountable in a common-sense, real-life approach.**

When your personality and approach with people push out practical common sense, you lose touch with the truth and what is really going on around you. When common sense is absent, there is a perception that you are not smart or even ignorant; perception, for some, IS their reality.

There are two things that cover up common sense and reveal ignorance. One we have previously discussed: *"Small-town thinking."* The second may be the biggest detriment to your overall success; admittedly or not, it is the ID or EGO.

The Power of the ID

Listen up, and listen well. Your mind costs you thousands of dollars a year either in lack of believability and imagination, small-town thinking, or EGO in the form of pride—the strongest negative emotion/feeling there is. Let me give you a common example of how pride reveals one's ignorance while pushing out common sense.

Common Sense and the Titanic

The thing that sank the Titanic before it even sailed was the fact that the engineers thought that the ship was unsinkable. Cockiness, naïveté, and maybe a little bit of denial pushed all forms of using common sense out the window, and then before they knew it, down they sank.

If you think that you are above reproach or your business is better than the rest, your business (ship) is already sinking and it will only be a matter of time before it's under water.

Ignorance is NOT Bliss

In the fitness training business, not knowing something is NOT bliss, but it is a money loser. One thing I like about fitness training is that every person is different. The exercises may be similar, but the people are challenge. This is why you have to teach on a common-sense level for them to get it and get results.

Reality, Relativity and Repetition

The more real you can be and more relative you can teach in modern times and in their language, the better, and this combined with a consistent over-and-over approach works best.

Money Tip- Reality does not bite when it comes to common sense. Education is great, but is worthless if you can't get people to relate to and understand what you are teaching.

Common Sense 101 Review

I guess another way you can describe common sense is: The more relatable you make teachable moments, the better results you will get out of your clients. Don't be ignorant or assume that your clients get everything you are telling or teaching them.

Attitude- Free your mind, and the rest will follow.
Theme- Acquiring cash is mental more than physical.
Tagline- The Creative Process to Prosperity.

VI

People 101

The "Art" of Motivating the Heart

People 101 Overview

Success is not measured in numbers on a chart, but is determined by the relationships you build. People really do put more importance on caring than knowing; miss that, and you will influence only yourself and not the world.

When dealing with people, being emotionally in tune goes much farther than intelligence. One size does not fit all, and assuming is a sure formula for failure. If you hide behind a piece of paper or degree, people will leave you, first emotionally and then physically. At the end of the day, knowing people and caring about your profession will win you more cash and relationships than trying to influence them through your past accomplishments. Master the *"Art"* of people, and the cash will be there for the asking.

21
The Art of "People" Training

Yes, training people is an art! I know that it may sound as though I do not believe in institutional education, but I most certainly do; it's a must in most cases. However, I cannot overstate the importance of great people skills. *This is the biggest demise of most fitness trainers; they think that a piece of paper makes them money. It does nothing other than get them a foot in the door. People make you money!*

The Art of People

Developing relationships with people requires a lot of things on your part. Understanding them and the role of fitness in their lives is crucial. People in general are not complicated; we just make them do things. Individuals want different things, but need basically the same things.

First, you must know how people tick and what their basic needs are in general. Each individual who comes to hire you wants certain needs and concerns met — make a note. Then insert the basic system of fitness to match their personality.

The Art of Assumption (NOT)

It makes me a little sick to discuss all of the mistakes I have made assuming peoples needs, what they can afford or not, and how long they will be a client. I have lost and left much money on the table because I assumed way too much! You have to just throw all assumptions out the door when it comes to people. Just follow your principles, beliefs and mission statement of your business, and let the cards fall where they may.

The Art of Giving Back

Give them more than they ask for, and they will return again and again. This sounds simple, but it's not always easy to do. However, it helps if you have this type of attitude. If you give more to them, they will continue to give back to you in money and referrals.

The Art of Knowing Your Audience

Fill a void or need, and give back as much as you can. That pretty much sums it up. But, you have to know your audience first. You have to know who and what you are dealing with. You can have the greatest of intentions and approach, but not have a clue as to the needs of the person. This takes more of a gut thing than book smarts.

22
EQ vs. IQ

Yes, success comes from intuition! Emotional Intelligence (EQ) — either you have it or you don't. Emotional intelligence is not the same thing as the "X" Factor. EQ is from the gut; IQ is from the classroom.

Intuition/Discernment

Intuition, by definition, is the act or faculty of knowing or sensing without the use of rational processes.

Discernment, by definition, is the act or process of exhibiting keen insight and good judgment.

I will be the first to admit that I am not the smartest person academically. Sure, I had a 3.5 GPA in the physical therapy school, but it was a real struggle. I'm not so sure how I received such high marks, to be honest. However, what I do know is that over the years I have proven time and time again my keen sense of awareness of people, predicting behaviors in the future.

Emotionally in Tune!

When mastering the art of people as it pertains to fitness training, achieving goals, balancing personalities and motivation, you HAVE to have some form of EQ. You have to be in tune with your client. (This is why I spend a large amount of time in my client orientation sessions.)

Lack of prudent judgment in the end will cost you clients and dollars and cents.

Greg Ryan

23
The Art of "Training" People

Yes, it's about how people tick! The secret of training people lies in four words: *encouragement, guidance, accountability, and responsibility.* None of these do any good unless you know the secrets to *"People Training,"* all of which we have discussed in earlier chapters.

To make money in the fitness training profession, you must incorporate not one, two, or three, but all of these areas in your business, every day with every client.

A Matter of Meaningful Importance

The order in which people view the importance of these areas may surprise you. **If you said accountability, responsibility, encouragement, and guidance, you are correct!** I'm willing to bet most of you thought otherwise.

Whether a person or client will ever admit it, studies show that people need and want responsibility, accompanied by accountability. Follow that up with guidance and a strategically placed word or encouragement, and you are well on your way. (I wish that it were that simple.)

A Matter of Balance

The *"Art"* of training people lies in the balancing of the four. Yes, I said *balance.* There will never be a time when one or more of the four components will not have to be addressed. Your goal is to juggle—or, more importantly, stay one step ahead of—the balancing act.

This is why learning the "Art" of people and how they tick is vital to your success in the fitness industry. This is why the X's and O's on a fitness chart or weight loss food plan are not the most important thing.

A Matter of Perspective

If you want to get the best results from your clients, you have to put yourself in their shoes. Understanding the situation from their perspective will make your job a little easier. We all have different histories and personalities that make the balancing act of training a daily challenge, to say the least.

A Matter of Need, Not Want

When it comes to training people, none of the above matters unless you follow through on what your client NEEDS, not what the clients wants. This will be a challenge from day one. Giving advice on what a client needs verses what he or she wants to hear may break a relationship and a financial agreement. This is why I mentioned this last, even though it is the most important of matters to attend to.

If you do these things, it develops a relationship that allows you to give the needed advice with a more open mind from your client. In the end, it still requires some confidence in the form of leadership. It also requires the right approach for that personality type.

24
Personality Type Programming

Yes, it's about personality! While everyone requires one or all three—accountability, motivation, and knowledge—these are just common elements to follow with each person. They will only take you so far without the right approach for that individual. **The right approach is determined by personality types, yet most trainers have not a clue regarding the importance of this.**

This may be the closet a fitness trainer will come to being a true psychologist. If you are good at what we are about to discuss, you are well on your way to being a RICH TRAINER.

One Size Does Not Fit All

One exercise program does fit everyone that comes through the door. More importantly, you cannot take one *approach* to everyone, either. Fitness trainers make this mistake over and over. While the exercises may be similar in nature, the approach should not be. This may only be able to be determined by your EQ. Your IQ or intellectual intelligence has no clue about people and their behaviors. IQ is more of a black-and-white, facts-driven, problem-solving way of thinking. EQ, on the other hand, is more intuitive and creative, with no boundaries, so to speak—more grey, if you will.

Exercise Programs- Keep it Real and Simple

While some exercise programs can be duplicated, for the majority, their progress will be short-lived in the long run.

Trainers give out or design the same program for many clients because it saves time and or energy. In the end, doing so will cost you money. Each exercise program should be customized to fit the client's needs, goals and lifestyle. Keep it simple, and keep it real.

Exercise programs and their success are only as good as designing the right approach, and this takes more than just talent. RICH TRAINERS understand that fitness training is more of an art than anything, and your canvas is a person's personality.

Behaviorist- *a person who specializes in the study of human behavior.* Much of what I am about to say is what the "X" Factor chapter of this book talks about. It's worth discussing it more in depth because it may be the biggest influence in you becoming RICH.

When it comes to exercise programming and implementing an accountability system, one type of approach does not fit all. Most trainers think that it does, and when their client does not respond, they blame it on the client.   There is a popular diet book called *Eat Right for Your Blood Type*. It teaches you how to eat for the particular blood type you have. Implementing weight loss and exercise programs is similar. If you want to be a successful and even RICH, you have to design programs to fit the individual's personality.

Personality Type Programming .

There are basically two types of personalities: *"A"* and *"B."* Each personality type views the world through different glasses. Their interaction with people, the way they communicate, and how they go about achieving things in life are basically opposing.

Type "A"

Strong-willed, straight shooter, task-oriented, and high expectations would describe an "A" type individual. An "A" type personality does not necessarily respond well with those of the opposing "B" personality. Frustration, awkwardness and impatience usually follow A's when dealing with B's. When it comes to designing and implementing fitness programs, A's are much easier to manage.

"A" type personalities love straightforward, goal- or task-oriented programs laid out in advance. They respect no-fluff, tell-it-like-it-is accountability. They hate wasting time and want to get the most "bang" for the buck. A's like more of a stern approach with a little encouragement mixed in from time to time.

Type "B"

Easygoing, people-pleaser, get-it-done-whenever, take-it-or-leave-it goals in life usually can describe a Type "B" personality. B types don't deal with A's very well; they feel intimidated and at times pushed into things. B types are a little more challenging in implementing programs.

"B" types take a more of a hands-on or passive approach. B's require encouragement more often with a common-sense, roundabout way of accountability. You cannot motivate them the same way as with an A. Just as all exercise charts do not fit every client, neither does the same approach fit each person and his or her personality.

Assuming Costs Money

My new client orientations are two hours long. Health history, expectations from each side, eating and psychological behavior reviews, and getting to know that individual's personality are all covered. You should avoid at all costs implementing a "B" type passive approach with an "A" type personality and vice versa; a "B" type will not respond well or not at all to an "A" approach.

In other words, if you are too laid back and lack accountability, an "A" type will view you as weak, wishy-washy and a waste of his or her money and time. On the other hand, if you get in the face of a "B" type by being too direct and stern, a he or she will run and quit because your approach is too abrasive.

My average client retention is over five years and at a pretty good price, because I learned early on the importance of matching my approach with their personalities.

A Balancing Act

If you want to be prosperous, you have got to understand and do the above. There's one other very important issue to address, however. Some fitness trainers may be great at exercise prescription, others good at dealing with and understanding either "A" or "B" type personalities on their own.

The **"Art"** of dealing with people when it comes to fitness training is in the daily *"Balancing Act."*

Balancing for Cash

If you have been in the fitness training business for any length of time, you know that every day is a new experience.

You may have five different people see you a day with five different personalities that can and will change on any given day. **This requires an extremely high level of intuition, emotional energy, confidence and faith in what you are doing.**

Maybe even more important is timing. You have got to know when, where and how to deal with both types of personalities every single day. Knowing how to mix encouragement and/or accountability with the cards you are dealt by each personality type is an *"Art."* In my opinion, this cannot be taught. **This, my friend, is the best description I have for the "X" Factor.**

Knowing how to mix encouragement and/or accountability with the cards you are dealt daily by each personality type is an "Art." In my opinion, this cannot be taught. This, my friend, is the best description I have for the "X" Factor.

Greg Ryan

25
Storytelling for Cash

Yes, it's about a story! *"People don't care how much you know as much as they want to know that you care."* The fitness training business is all about people and relationships.

I'm not trying to be harsh, but if you hide behind the X's and O's on a chart or your status/ego-stroking Ph.D. in exercise physiology, guess what? Your new client will become an old one very quickly. If all you care about is the paycheck, put it in savings, because you probably won't get many more from them. And if you think that one motivational speech will inspire for life, I suggest that you read the timeless book *How to Win Friends and Influence People*.

Connecting Equals Cash

No matter if it's networking with professionals or the clients themselves — building relationships is the key to wealth. This can only be accomplished if you believe in your cause and in the welfare of the people. When cash becomes more of the motive than caring, your financial well may dry up sooner rather than later.

One of the reasons I have not had to spend as much *money* on outside advertising is because I spend more *time* building relationships — time in the beginning very well spent. As a result, my client retention has spanned an average of five to eight years.

Storytelling for Money

One of the best ways of connecting with people is by telling stories they can relate to. Being a good listener is the first important quality you must have; the second is *storytelling.*

If you can tell a true story of a third person, or a personal yet aboveboard one of your own, they will most likely connect with you on a deeper level. When people can relate, they will do better. Pie-in-the-sky stuff never works long-term. Storytelling also gets your point across more effectively without putting people on the defensive. Follow-up questions are always good after a story, as well. This builds bonds of respect in the end and creates cash retention.

People 101 Review

People are attracted to caring more than knowing. EQ reaches hearts more than IQ. Every person is different, so your approach must be, as well. Personalities are unique, so you may have to tell a few relatable stories. Master the *"Art"* of people, and the cash will be there for the taking.

Attitude- Making money in fitness is about people, not charts.
Theme- Learn how each client ticks, and customize the approach accordingly.
Tagline- The Art of Motivation Lies in the People.

EQ is more lucrative than IQ.

VII

Leadership 101

The "Purpose" of the Plan

Leadership 101 Overview

You are paid to lead. You are expected to pave the way. With no spine, you will crumble. Confidence, love, transparency and actions are the strength of good leadership. Are these learned? I'm not sure. Can you develop them over time with experience? Probably so.

Leadership is not always easy. It requires hope, belief in what you are doing, and faith in the future. It requires saying no when every part about you wants to say yes. It oftentimes goes against the norm of those around you, and it most likely will have some form of consequences to follow. In the end, however, you, others around you, and this world will be better off for such actions. It is then up to you to continue to push forward, even if the world pushes back.

26
Lead with Confidence

Yes, leading takes a spine! *Doing the right thing, even when it's not popular!* I have always tried to live by those words. It's not easy and requires guts, faith, foresight and confidence. No matter their age, current health status or even level of optimism, people hire you to lead even when times get tough.

Strong Leadership

Leadership comes in different forms and is one of the hardest things for trainers to possess. For me, this was and is a delicate balance of business, tough love and compassion. And you'd better know when to use each. Strong leadership requires humility, honesty and good hearing. It is not competitive in nature and possesses no pride. It means believing in someone even when they do not have confidence in themselves.

Lead with Confidence

Leadership demands confidence. Holding people to their goals takes a willingness to let go. Having a belief that what you are asking or even demanding of them is the right thing for them, even if they cannot see it at the time.

Lead with Guts

Having the strength to walk away from a check takes guts. It takes a belief system that you are doing the right thing. It also takes a little bit of....

Lead with Foresight

You have to know where you are going. Business and personal mission statements help determine that. To make it as a trainer, you have to be a dreamer. You have to inspire yourself more than anyone. You have to have the foresight of your future, or you will fail.

Lead without Confusion

Teach, test, and tell the truth in a loving, straightforward manner. Teach your clients daily. Test them once in a while on what they have learned. Tell the truth no matter what, and lead by backing everything up to teach with logic, reason, common sense, and real stories.

27
Lead with Love

Yes, it's about empathy! *It's not about you* when it comes to the success of your <u>clients.</u> *It IS all about you* when it comes to the success of your <u>business.</u> Remember this quote?

Leadership is only as good as how much your clients respect you. Respect is not given; it's earned through caring. They don't have to love you, but they must respect you if they are going to succeed. Let's face it: Fitness training is a relationship thing. And in any relationship, the two most important aspects are love and respect. You can love someone and not respect them, and you can also respect someone and not love them. But if you want both to grow, they must both feed on each other.

If you <u>respect</u> your clients, they will in turn grow to <u>love</u> you and what you stand for. If you <u>love</u> what you do, others will grow to <u>respect</u> what you do. If you truly care about (love) people, you will respect yourself.

Gaining respect is a lot harder than losing it. You can lose their trust very quickly. One way is by being a......

Hypocrisy

Be very careful not to say one thing and do another. And be consistent with whatever you teach or say. People may not like what you have to say, but if you say it consistently, they will respect you at least.

Empty Words

Do as I say, not as I do! You may be surprised by how many trainers have this thought pattern.

They may not say it or even consciously think it, but something doesn't line up. What they are teaching and doing themselves may be miles apart.

I have had numerous people in my life whom at one time I looked up to and respected. After a while, I noticed that their words were not aligning with their actions. What they had said before was starting to lose its influence. In other words, I lost respect for them and what they were saying; they were empty words to me — in one ear and out the other.

Your clients don't have to love you to succeed, but they do need to respect you.

28
Lead with Silence

Yes, leadership requires listening! Leadership takes on many different forms, including some you may not think it would. Let's be real: You don't have to have iron man fitness levels, a pencil-thin waistline or bulging biceps to be a good fitness trainer. However:

"Make your actions speak so loudly that what you say cannot be heard."

Lead in Silence

One thing that I have really tried hard to do over the last three decades is be in the best shape I could be. My hardbody days were over early on, but I still wanted to be in good shape. It wasn't any easier for me, either. Still, I just felt like I would have been a hypocrite if I let myself go.

Lower Body Fat, Higher Income

I did an interesting study in the 1990s while living in Los Angeles: I graphed my body fat to my income levels. The findings were enlightening.

For three years I monitored my body fat levels and my income levels. What was interesting was that they were directly related; the lower my body fat, the higher my income. The two things I observed were my confidence level and the perception of me from others. Subconsciously I felt better about myself, which translated into dollars. The other thing was that people assumed that I must know something about fitness.

You don't have to have two percent body fat or bulging biceps or be a marathon runner, but you need to try to be in the best shape you can. If you do that, then you can say a lot without uttering a word. I cannot tell you how much money I have made living by this leadership principle alone.

Transparency

Many times, clients just need to relate to someone who shares the same challenges with weight that they have. When people can relate, they let their walls down and listen more to your advice. Be honest with them; share some of your own challenges with fitness. However, that should be as far as it goes. People will end up respecting you more and taking to heart what you are teaching them.

29
Lead with Boundaries

Yes, leading is about limits! *Boundaries* are limits, rules or guidelines that are enforced by you. Most trainers do NOT have the confidence to enforce boundaries. Why? Well, you may lose them if you make them angry. They have the power, since they wrote the check.

If you have children, you will understand this point. Adults, just as it is with children, may not initially like having guidelines or rules imposed on them, but deep down they want the structure. If you can remember that, enforcing boundaries by holding them accountable to their goals becomes a little easier.

You will be tested, I promise you, so you have to be consistent. The minute you are not and let a client slide, you lose the respect from them and the authority. If you are just in the business for the money, you will never master this art of training. Thus, you will never be wealthy. There are mainly three reasons you are hired as fitness trainer: encouragement, knowledge and accountability.

Motivation/Encouragement

Every human being needs and wants encouragement. If you give too much, however, it enables them; if you give them too little, it never empowers them—a fine line to follow, for sure.

Knowledge

To be a successful trainer, this may be one of the most important areas to master. And I am not so sure that it's teachable. If you have any leadership skills, they will be tested with this one.

"Make your actions speak so loudly that what you say cannot be heard."

30
Lead with Accountability

Yes, it mostly comes down to accountability! When it comes to leadership and success in this business, the area of accountability is vital.

Fitness training is similar to raising kids. There is a balancing act to conduct every day. Whether people say it or not, they hire trainers for a *reason* to exercise. Whether they like it or not, people want structure, rules and boundaries. Needless to say, that does not guarantee that they will like them or even follow them. Depending on the age of the person, it will determine your approach and how well they receive such guidelines. At the end of the day, in order for clients to succeed they need to take responsibility in their lives and be held accountable for the daily choices they make; this is what they hire you for.

There are mainly three reasons a person hires a fitness trainer: *knowledge, motivation and accountability.* In what order of importance do you think they are with most people? If you said that knowledge or motivation is number one, guess what: You are wrong! Whether they say they do or not, the majority of individuals enter your doors for a *reason* to exercise— someone to answer to.

They don't teach a course in college on holding people accountable, do they? And unless you are a psychology major, you don't learn how people are motivated, either. **The success of your fitness training career lies in your ability to hold clients accountable when required and motivated when needed. Knowledge is just means to an end.**

Now, you medical and classroom types may not like to hear that, but thirty years in the trenches has taught me that, not an anatomy book.

Accountability

Accountability, by definition, is *taking or being assigned responsibility for something that you have done or something you are supposed to do.*

The bottom line is that people hire trainers to hold them accountable to their goals. They may change their minds once they start, though, because it's harder than they thought. Still, in the end they don't have the discipline to hold themselves to their aspirations, so they need a person to answer to.

Here is the challenge: *"They pay you!"* How can you truly hold one accountable who, in the end, holds all of the power? The answer is: You have to. This funny thing is, grown-ups are just like children when it comes to accountability. They want it deep down. They may not like the process, but in the end they love the structure. I am shocked that the more I hold a person accountable, the longer they stay with me as clients. Why? They are getting results. However, accountability does not work unless you have......

Responsibility

Responsibility, by definition, is *the quality or state of being responsible: as a: moral, legal, or mental accountability b: reliability, trustworthiness.*

Holding a client responsible **for** their goals is very different from holding them accountable **to** their goals.

Responsibility means giving something away. You have to relinquish control and give it to your clients. All you are having to do is manage them—easier said than done. This takes a lot of energy, and has a lot to do with people skills.

Boundary Follow-through

Change your mindset about boundaries

This is the first step because if you can't do this, everything else will be unsuccessful. Boundaries serve to protect relationships, not harm them; you're not being mean. For the co-dependent folks who are reading this post, this is going to be challenging for you. But I'm here to tell you that if you don't learn how to set boundaries in your business, you will find yourself continually taken advantage of and stressed.

Create the boundary

Decide where you're going to place the garden hose.

Remove your emotions

Don't allow yourself to be sucked into an emotional conversation. Stick to the facts. (See #4.)

Have the conversation.

Here's a sample script you can use.

(Take responsibility.) "I know for the past few months I've let you…"

(The business case) "After analysing my business, I see that I need to…"

(Set the boundary) "So from now on, I will… and I need you to…"

Reinforce the boundary

You're going to have to reinforce your boundaries. They will be pushed and tested. Stand strong.

Ways to Enforce your Business Boundaries

Last-minute Requests – Sometimes your clients may call on you for last-minute help, which in a service business isn't a problem. The trouble is when last-minute becomes the norm and you can't manage your project load because you are constantly rushing for the chronic offenders who just can't seem to get it together. Charge an additional fee if you can't say no.

Managing Your Client Roster – Sometimes it seems scary to put a new client on hold until you have time in your schedule, but it's critical from a quality (and sanity) control perspective.

Scope Creep – More often than not, as you get into a project, you discover more ways you can help your client. A little extra here, a little bit there, and before you know it, you are doing double the work.

THE BOUNDARY FIX: Know when to put on the brakes when it comes to doing extra work. "That is beyond the original scope of the work and will require additional fees. I will send over an estimate of the additional amount required to complete those tasks."

Rules of Engagement – It's ENTIRELY up to you how you want to work with your clients.

THE BOUNDARY FIX: "Before getting started, we require a signed proposal and a deposit." And nothing (and I mean NOTHING) gets done until that step is complete.

After-hours Work Calls – Just because your clients work late at night, on the weekends or what seems like 24/7, doesn't mean that you need to. Be clear with what hours you are available to take business calls and respond to e-mail.

Money Tips- Your success as a fitness trainer comes down to holding clients accountable and empowering them with responsibilities.

Leadership 101 Review

Being a good leader requires guts, a spine and faith. In the fitness business you are paid to lead, no matter what. Holding an adult in this world accountable for his or her actions goes against the grain, and at times is not politically correct. So, what? Many times, leadership is shown in just listening or tough love, each one in a timely manner.

Attitude- Leadership requires conviction and tough love.
Theme- It's not what they want, but what they need.
Tagline- A Purpose to the Plan.

VIII
Marketing 101
The "Power" through Leveraging

Marketing 101 Overview

Work smart, not hard, we must. Accomplish more with less, we strive for. Duplicating our time, we pay for. Promoting our brand, you long for.

Marketing is a never-ending, energy-draining, time-consuming, money-sucking necessity in life and business. From our childhood, we have been conditioned to sell ourselves to others and the world. Today, the art of marketing seems too be about two things: branding and leveraging; develop a signature name or trademark, and somehow position yourself to be more effective with less. I.e.... the Internet.

Whatever your goals and the means you use to reach them are, a consistent system of promotion is the key. Like with a lot of things, it's not rocket science, but it does require discipline, dedication and perseverance.

31
Branding You

Yes, your identity is your Brand. *Branding-* The process involved in creating a unique name and image for a product in the consumer's mind.

The goal for any company or individual owning a business is to develop an identity or *Brand*—something that others remember you or the business by. This requires consistent habits over a period of time, and must be sustained at a certain level as long as one is in business. Fitness training is no different: Develop a name, image and reputation about you and your business; this takes time.

You the Brand

Like I said, "Yes, it's a business, and yes, it's personal." Here's where it gets personal. Your brand is your identity. A former boss once said to me, *"You are always on stage."* In other words, you are always being watched by someone: peers, associates, family, potential clients, and those you don't even realize are watching. You can work extremely hard, and in a moment wipe it out with some stupid decision, action or statement. Everything about you is being branded on the minds of the world. Life is a mirror, and your brand is being reflected all over the place.

Without saying anything, your Brand should say all there is to know about you. Here are things to ask yourself when developing a brand:

-How do you want others to see you?
-What do you want others to first think when they see you and your logo and image?

-What does your brand do for others?
-What does your brand say about you?

Consistency Pays

When developing a brand name or image, you must always be consistent in your marketing. If you change things around, it will be confusing. The market does not like complicated messages. Once you have decided on an image or a logo, mission statement and philosophy, do not change it. Years down the road, sure, but not in the near future. Do not be wishy-washy; the world can see it—the customer can feel it, and you cannot stop it when that starts.

32
The Pied Piper Principle

Yes, it's about getting your brand out! The goal of marketing is get the word out, create a brand that's memorable, and what?

The Pied Piper Principle

The money is in your following. You have to create a wave of followers. If you can get one to follow you, getting a thousand is no different. So, how to you get the Pied Piper to play and the rats to follow? LOL!

Good Service

This may go without saying, but if you give good customer service, you will have a following—it's simple.

Good Education

Educate! People follow those who give them good information or content that they can incorporate in their daily lives. Always—and I mean always—try to teach by supplying useful information.

Good Content through Technology

I learned early on that to be successful on the Internet, and specifically blogs, you have to write good content. With technology, the distribution system is there; now you have to give them the above—good content to educate.

Good Business Principles

Whether you realize it or not, people can tell what you stand for by how you act, what you believe in, how you treat them, and how you conduct business. People want to be led, and if you can sell them on your actions and what you believe in, then they will continue to follow you as long as you do that.

Good Consistency

Creating a following is not an overnight accomplishment, especially on the Internet. You have to be consistent every day and in everything you do and say. The thing to remember is this: **"You can lose followers easier than getting them!"**

33
Leverage Your Brand

Kathy Smith was a very gracious person when I worked for her years ago. She was also a marketing guru. During the early 1990s, I managed a health club in Santa Monica, California called <u>Mezzeplex.</u> During that time, we became great friends.

One month out of the year, Kathy would dedicate time to the making of a fitness video. In her world, it was all about duplication. Film a video, dub it, and sell as many of them as possible. Every time someone watched it, she was working. She made millions. Not bad for a month's worth of work a year. Kathy taught me the power of duplication. Sooner or later, you have to find a system of leveraging your time and brand.

Leverage- Positional advantage; power to act effectively.

Time in a bottle

Do you know that the only thing this world cannot create and manufacture is time? With technology, it is easier than ever to leverage your time and knowledge. Everything I do, every word I write on paper, has the ability to be duplicated or leveraged. You may be reading this while I am golfing, sleeping, eating, or out on the lake with a drink in my hand; all the while, I am working as I play. Money or time, it doesn't matter — the power is in the leveraging of it.

It's not about you when it comes to the success of your <u>clients.</u> *It IS all about you* when it comes to the success of your <u>business.</u>

34
Social Media Marketing 101

Yes, marketing is about the Internet! The world has changed, and so have the ways and means of developing a brand for you or your business. Rich people find so-called rivers of money, and they swim in it daily. If you are going to be successful in marketing your company, you have to find the currents of cash cyberspace to get your brand in front of the specific markets you want.

About the time you finally learn a trend of social media, it changes to something else. Find something that works for you and stick with it. For me at this point in my career, it's book writing and selling my knowledge. For you it may be a particular niche market of clients you want to train, or promotion of your training business, or a product you created.

"Synergize" Your Brand

Synergizing your brand is the goal! The whole is only as good as the sum of its parts, you must remember. While each tool of social media is ways of letting the world know who you are, the goal is to connect them in a way that creates momentum, like a tidal wave. Hopefully, you get to a point where you can stop it if you wanted to.

The secret behind these tips is to allow you to create a **"social media synergy"** that totals a sum far greater than the individual parts. Some of these tips are basic, but at the very least they can serve as a checklist that may assist you in synergizing your online presence and bringing traffic and viewers to your global digital properties.

Here are a few ways I have used social media outlets to promote my products, services and brand in a synergistic way. It will not happen overnight, but keep at it, and the little ripple will grow into a tidal wave!

Blogging

Blogs, while time-consuming, are one of the easiest platforms to create a brand name for you and your company. Nothing is more influential than great, consistent information that helps a selected market. And nothing creates a more dedicated following of people who may buy a product from you in the future, either. Personally, I have four blogs that I post on every week. If you are serious about social media marketing, create a blog and write. Here are a few tips to consider if you do:

1. Produce inspiring, educational and awesome content that is so compelling that people want to share it; this is the foundation of your marketing.

2. Write regularly and consistently. People will then come and visit regularly and keep coming back because they know that it will be new and topical.

3. Write a headline that makes people want to read the rest of your article.

4. Use "list" posts regularly. They may be a bit passé for some, but they work and tend to get passed around online.

5. Place Retweet, Facebook, and LinkedIn buttons on your blog.

6. Include a Facebook "like box" near the top right side of the blog so that people can "like" your Facebook page

even while they are on your blog.

7. Make it easy for people to subscribe via e-mail (e-mail marketing may be perceived as old school, but it works big-time!).

8. Provide "subscribe" buttons so that people can follow you on your other web properties (Facebook, Twitter, LinkedIn, etc.).

9. Provide a subscription button via RSS so that people can have your posts pushed to them in their "Google Reader" account after they are published.

10. When you have a great idea, go straight to your "add new" button, and write the headline and save it as a draft, or write it down before you forget it.

Creating a following will not happen overnight, but keep at it. Sooner or later, you will create a brand for yourself by blogging.

Twitter

To tweet or not to tweet? I used to think that tweeting was for the birds. I thought that it was for those who had nothing better to do; boy, I was wrong! It has turned out to be one of the best moneymaking social media tools I have. Everything that I do is linked to Twitter (richtrianer1). Here are some tips:

1. Acquire Twitter followers; quantity is important.

2. Engage and develop Twitter followers within your niche.

3. Share the content of influential Twitter people.

4. Automate the tweeting of other bloggers' content that you trust.

5. Tweet regularly and consistently the posts of other influential bloggers in your topic category.

6. Automate the retweeting of your great content so that it is not forgotten and buried in the archives.

7. When tweeting your posts, include # tags that deliver the tweet.

8. Share valuable content in your own voice.

9. Use keywords in your tweets.

10. Share links to useful content.

11. Use search features to discover what your clients want.

12. Connect with the right people, and tweet with them.

13. Use a classic icebreaker.

14. Cultivate relationships.

15. Engage your audience.

16. Be helpful.

17. Transparency lends credibility.

18. Use hashtags to create and curate conversations around your brand.

19. Share links back to your website for list building.

20. Tweet links to your blog more often.

Don't abuse the media, but be consistent with meaningful, useful content; this helps the brand.

Facebook

Facebook! Ever get tired of hearing that word? It's very unique phenomenon: People visit it not for any particular reason, but to find a reason to stay. Knowing that, make them have a reason to stay on your pages. In the future, it may be the best free advertisement you can get. Here are some tips:

1. Update your Facebook "page" with your blog posts immediately after publishing them.

2. Provide content and links on your Facebook page that will make them want to share and "like" your updates.

3. Include Twitter in your menu (this is available as a standard setting on your Facebook fan page).

4. Run polls using the standard Facebook "Question" feature (above the "Write something" box) to engage your audience and involve them.

5. Link to your Facebook page in your e-mail newsletter.

6. Run a competition on Facebook.

7. Use a reveal tab that is set up as your landing page that provides access to unique content; this could be a video, some content, or even a voucher.

8. Respond to all comments on your Facebook page in a timely fashion.

Facebook is a necessary thing to do in building a brand for yourself. It's free advertising for you at this point. Synergy-wise, everything is linked and posted to all my Facebook pages.

LinkedIn

LinkedIn has been a great social media tool for me when connecting with those in the industry and promoting my books. Here are some tips that I have learned:

1. Use all three websites or links that LinkedIn allows in your profile (these can point to your website, blog and Facebook).

2. Make your LinkedIn profile "public" in your settings.

3. Pose questions in the Q&A section of LinkedIn with links to your possible answer as a post link.

4. Setup a LinkedIn profile for your blog (not just your personal profile).

5. Integrate your Slideshare into your LinkedIn account using the "Add an Application" button at the bottom right of your home page.

6. Integrate your blog post feed into your LinkedIn account using the "Add an Application" button at the bottom right corner of your home page.

7. Add your Twitter feed into your LinkedIn account using the "Add an Application" button.

LinkedIn is about developing longer-term relationships with those in your profession and industry; it's not about selling them a product, at least up front. Don't abuse the system, but definitely post and get involved in discussion groups.

YouTube

YouTube may be responsible for more success stories than anything over the last ten years. Those who never would have been noticed, now have the ways and means to do so.

1. Interview influential people in your topic category on video, and post them to YouTube.

2. Include your website/blog link in your profile.

3. Automate sharing after posting (available under "Account Settings" then "Activity Sharing," then choose the social accounts, and as a minimum select Facebook and Twitter (Reader, Orkut and MySpace are also able to be enabled).

4. Write a headline that is "keyword"-rich for your industry and niche.

5. Write a tempting and teasing headline that makes the potential viewer want to "hit" the play button.

6. Place a link to your blog at the beginning of each description for each video. Make sure that you write a description that includes keywords and an inviting description. Include keyword tags for each video.

Google+

From what I've seen and heard, Google+ is really blowing up right now. I think one of the main reasons for this is that GFC is going away, and Wordpress and other non-blogger users are going to want to stay connected. Google+ could be the glue that holds us all together. I think it could possibly become better than GFC/Google Reader because in my opinion, it's easier to navigate than those other gadgets.

However, use it on a regular basis and you will like it even more, as the search results are a lot more relevant. Below are some of the features that set **Google+** apart.

Media

Media files added on <u>Google+</u> are distinctively interesting and appealing to the eyes. You are able to view photos either in large sizes or small ones with ease and convenience. The photos look realistically attractive, a feature that many online users seem to like. You can zoom in and out easily without difficulty, and the photo does not blur. It is even a lot better than when you integrate your photos on other sites. Besides, Google+ will provide updates once you check on their visuals.

Mobile

Without ample time to spare setting up your computer, the only convenient gadget that you can use is your mobile phone. Through applying for the necessary applications on your phone, you can already view photos without setbacks and have a greater and wider communication range on Huddles.

Phone Apps

While this may not be considered a social media thing, the customized phone app in connection with Itunes is a must for your brand. Again, keep in mind that it's about convenient information gathering from your followers. The more tools they have to gather your stuff, the more likely they will follow you and eventually buy your product or service. You can design your apps with any of the social media sites that we have talked about on it.

Benefits

Here are some of the benefits of having your own app for your fitness business:

Promotes your brand
It maximizes your approach to your market
Cost-effective
It keeps you viral and recognized quickly
People connect to you anywhere

The Goal

The goal is simple: Be able to communicate with as many people anywhere, anytime.

Podcasting

Another media avenue worth mentioning is *podcasting*. Podcasts are audio recordings of anything at practically any length. The future of information will be visual and audio, not text. So, to succeed in cyberspace, you will have to adapt to the system, and podcasting is part of that.

I am currently converting all of my books into audio form, and within a few months, all of my blog posts will either be podcasting or video—no text. Today, I can be on the beach with my iPhone, recording a podcast of some useful training information for you, hit a button and automatically post an audio recording to my blog post—just like that!

Podcasting for Pay

Your podcasts can also make you money. Pick a subject of value, record it, post it, and link it to a PayPal system, and you are finished. It's that simple.

The Goal

The goal with podcasting is to connect with each individual as personably and often as possible. When they can hear a person's voice, they will tend to take that person more seriously. It's human nature.

Podcasting and Clients

Podcasting can be a great tool for client retention. The more you help clients with their concerns, the better. Podcasting can act like a virtual trainer. Never hesitate to put down a recording of something and e-mail it to people. They will love that—it shows that you can do it.

Writing for Money

Social media can be in just about any form. For me, right now it's in any form of writing and audio. For you, it may be something different.

Writing for Cash

One of my goals back in the beginning was to get paid for my knowledge; little did I know that I could get paid so easily with the way technology was headed.

I've gotten paid for every bit of knowledge I put on paper or on a podcast—someway, somehow. All I had to do was write good stuff and ask for money.

Newsletters, corporations, gym franchises, weight loss centers, hometown schools... You name it, I would write for them—a great way to build your reputation and brand.

I might add that my knowledge was also linked to all of my social media sites for further income and branding.

Books

Anyone can write something and put it into a book form these days. You don't need a big-time publisher to do so. Book writing, whether you consider yourself a "real" author or not, gives you more credibility in the marketplace. And so:

Everything created must be synergized.

Speaking for Money

Anything I write, I speak about. Speaking, lecturing, motivational... Whatever you want to call it is up to you. I call it another income stream. Most hate to speak in front of people; which is fine with me, because then my value goes up even more. If you want to make money in a short period of time, learn to talk in front of people; make it informative, educational and inspirational.

Storytellers

The good speakers tell stories. Great speakers hook people in by getting them to relate to the stories they are talking about. If you want to make money speaking, tell stories—true ones. Even ones you have personally experienced. **Humility breeds familiarity, which attracts money.**

Speaker Branding

Once you get a comfortable speaking, find a niche and milk it for all it's worth. Make a name for yourself. I don't think there is anything more influential than making a name or brand for yourself as an expert speaker in your field.

Marketing 101 Review

Marketing and branding are a necessity in the fitness training business. Work smart or waste cash—not easy to predetermine. The art is in the *leveraging*. The power is in your **brand**. It's not rocket science, but it does require discipline, dedication and perseverance.

The key is to not forget the best way of building relationships, while at the same time not being left behind in today's social media world and technology. Marketing is about creating a brand and a following of that brand, and at the same time leveraging your brand in a way that all works together, building momentum like a title wave.

Attitude- Marketing an Identity
Theme- Leverage Your Brand
Tagline- The Power of Brand Leveraging

Know the goal, know your role, and keep the picture in your sights!

IX

Nutrition 101

The "Influence" of the Role Player

Nutrition 101 Overview

True, we are not dietitians, but there is no denying that food plays a vital role in the fitness trainer's profession. Can we educate? Sure. Can we solve all issues? No. In recognition of that, the big picture must never be lost. It is not the job of the trainer to micromanage or confuse, but to encourage and educate through good, sound nutrition practices. Our purpose lies more in teaching awareness and instilling accountability than anything.

You want to make money from the nutrition side of things, make them aware, hold them accountable and feed them supplements.

35
The Goal

What is the goal of a fitness trainer when it comes to implementing nutrition into a plan? Each trainer will have a different answer. That's fine; just never lose sight of the fact that there is a goal.

All or Nothing

Implementing food and behavior change into a program is most challenging, to say the least. In order for the client to succeed, follow-through must happen on both sides — yours and theirs. To accomplish this, you must first decide if money is more important than the client. What do I mean by that?

All of your talents will come down to this: Either you stick to your principles, knowledge and guidelines, or you allow the client to dictate the results. If they do, they will not succeed when it comes to food and weight loss. If money is more important to you, then you will allow them to control your goal. But what if you are afraid that they will leave you if you push too hard? Well, so then they do — unless the money, like I said, is more important to you.

So, I ask you again: *"What is your goal?"* Is it to make money, or to pacify your clients?

You have to have an all-or-nothing goal, or in the end they will not meet their goals and you will look like you are not doing your job. The first thing you must do when advising a client is to know your goal. The second is.....

Know your role, and roll with it!

36
The Role Player

Know your role! You've got the goal; now, the client must know what to expect and who does what. Each piece of the puzzle has a role that needs to be stated up front.

State Your Role

You are not a dietitian or nutritionist; do not claim to be, and state that up front with everyone you work with. Your role is that of a guidance counselor on food, vitamins and supplements. Now, how you do that varies with each person. In my world, there are two roles to play: a *Teacher* and an *Implementer*.

The Teacher- Awareness

What is the role of the teacher? Well, just like it states, you teach. The first job of the educator is to make a person aware of everything involved.

Awareness- The state or ability to perceive, to feel, or to be conscious of events, objects or sensory patterns.

The *Teacher's* role in your client's life is getting him or her to become aware of what he or she is eating, how much, and what the behavior patterns are. Good luck on this one. This will take some patience, guts, and many teachable moments. Becoming aware of one's habits is always the first and hardest step to take, but it is necessary.

The Implementer – Accountability

It's the hardest of all—holding your clients accountable, that its!

Accountability - The obligation of an individual or organization to account for its activities, accept responsibility for them, and to disclose the results.

Truthful, Direct Orientations

Why do I have two-hour orientations with potential clients? To make sure that they know what to expect from me and what I expect from them, and this includes holding their feet to the fire by being accountable to their goals, not mine.

The *"only"* way to succeed as a trainer is to follow through on implementing your and the client's goals through accountability—period.

Tough Love

In order for this whole nutrition thing to succeed, it will require from you day in and day out, two words: **"Tough Love."**

The money is in tough love!

37
The Big Picture

Yes, food is an *"Attitude"* as much as it is counting calories; maybe even more so. You always have to look at food from a larger perspective. As stated before, a fitness trainer's purpose is more in the follow-through than in the food itself. It's a lot easier to do that when you keep a larger perspective in mind. Keeping the big picture in mind does not mean that you have to be a dietitian. You can educate and encourage while at the same time, rather than confuse or complicate.

Caught in the Weeds

Yes, counting calories is necessary in the end, but don't get too hung up on them. You can get bogged down in the weeds and never get out if you are not careful. In other words, the client may think that it becomes too much of a job and quit.

Emotional Connections

In most cases, eating behaviors are due to deeper issues that require a person with a little higher pay grade, like a psychologist. Again, know your role, acknowledge that there are emotions behind the behavior, and admit when the issue is deeper than you can handle. The goal is to change the behavior, so why worry who helps you?

A Matter of Balance

If you push too hard, deprivation steps in. Encourage too little, and perseverance gives in. In other words, your job as a trainer with food and clients is a challenge, to say the least.

Changing one's food habits is a long process. With too many boundaries, people rebel; with not enough guidelines, they lose hope and confidence.

Play the percentages.

Sometimes you can get a little too detailed in teaching and implementing, especially when dealing with food, behaviors and clients. There's nothing wrong with covering your bases, but too much detail can overwhelm a person. I've found this to work best for me.....

Play the percentages

In other words, don't lose sight of the big picture here. Do not get too hung up on micromanaging; help your clients learn the percentage of types of foods—not always a calorie issue. If you get down in the weeds too much, you will get bogged down and lose sight of the goal.

In the end, your success percentages will go up as well as your pocketbook if you play the bigger percent or attitude game.

38
The Pen Power

When it comes to food counseling, there may be no better way to do your job than with a pen and paper.

I cannot express to you the power a pen and paper have or how it really works, but it does. It definitely makes one aware of their eating habits and in some way holds them accountable; numbers don't lie. Some will just call it journaling.

Journaling

When clients write things down, their words become magical. And I don't mean selective wordage; I mean everything.

A journal takes on two roles for me when dealing with food and people: awareness and emotional behavior. We already spoke about them just acknowledging what they eat, but then you have to speak of "why."

Emotional "Roller Coaster"
This is a very tricky part for a fitness trainer. Again, know your role. Do not claim to be a dietitian or a registered psychologist. I have never claimed to be either, but over the years I have become pretty darn good at the psychology part of fitness training.

When people journal, they become aware of their behavior. The next step is to help them become aware of the **"why's"** of that type of behavior.

I don't really think that you have to be a full-fledged psychologist to do this. It only requires a little common sense, in my opinion. If you can connect an eating pattern and a behavior with an emotion or feeling, you can start helping a client change his or her ways of eating. Either way, through you or a registered psychologist, it really doesn't matter; a journal is a necessary tool.

Journals, while a thorn in a client's side, are money in your pocket.

39
Programming for Personality

Yes, food and success are about personality! Food, more than even exercise, is a personality programming issue. If you are going to help the individual out for the long run, you have to match the food program with the person's personality. Here is where I may lose a few trainers, but stay with me on this one. You may have to compromise your strict structure in order for the client to reach his or her goals.

Program for personality.

This is by far the most important part to learn in fitness training, no matter if it's exercise or food. You have to match the approach with the personality.

I don't care what weight loss or nutrition program one uses from my list, as long as one follows through with it. Your client will fail in the end if the approach does not match his or her personality.

Here is a short list of the most popular weight loss programs over the last fifteen years. Each one has its good and not-so-good points. Sure, they can be modified a little for your and the client's preferences, but as a trainer, don't be too anal retentive on doing it YOUR way; be flexible in this area. The more the client likes the approach, the more success he or she will have. Remember: manage, not micromanage.

Program Names	Theme of Program
Jenny Criag-	Portion Control- Convenience
Weight Watchers-	Portion Control- Accountability
Nutri-System-	Portion Control - Prepared Meals
South Beach-	Higher Protein- Low Carbohydrate
Sugar Busters-	Low Carbohydrates- No Sugar
Doctor Phil-	Behavior Modification

You may add more to the list, but the mindset is still the same: Match the program's approach with the client's mindset.

Nutrition 101 Overview

Implementing nutritional counseling is a vital component of a fitness trainer's job and the success of a client. Know your goal, role, and path, as well as personality of the client. Approach that with a big-picture attitude, and money will follow.

Attitude- The big picture is best; micromanaging hinders success.

Theme- Teach awareness, and enforce accountability.

Tagline- Never underestimate your role.

Your success as a fitness trainer comes down to holding clients accountable and empowering them with responsibilities.

X
Gym Owner 101

Gym Owner Overview

I write this from two points of view: the owner, and the fitness trainer. The goal is for you to see both sides of the coin and come up with a happy middle ground understanding.

Owner's Mission: *Increase the money, and decrease the turnover.* Good or bad economy, it matters not. Good or bad staffing — that matters a lot. As with clients, getting trainers is easier than keeping them. Getting good trainers is more challenging.

The trick is to balance what the service market price will bear, and what is fair in dividing that fee between the house and the trainer — an individual decision, at best. Can it be done? Sure, but we need to address it from both sides of the equation.

Trainer's Mission: Make as much money and get as much experience as one can.

So, the goal is to create a win-win from both sides. Here are some things for both sides to think about.

Part 1
The Gym Owner's Viewpoint

"Think Short-term with Incentives"

The profit is hidden in the motives!

39
Profit Margins

Profit margin! That's what it's about. You and I know that, but fitness trainers don't and could care less—so they should, to a point.

Margins

Margins are comparisons of sorts. Profit margins are financial statements that compare a business's gross income with its total expenses. The remaining amount is the working profit or capital. Profit margins are established in the business plan stages before anything. Margins are never the same month to month, so financial planners for companies will establish a range in which to operate.

The Overall Goal

The goal is for the margins to be higher rather than lower. The thing to understand is that higher gross income does not mean higher profit. Both income and expenses will vary monthly.

Training Department Goal

In order to reach the overall goal, each department has the same idea: Cut costs and increase cash flow. Owners really only make money when trainers make money.

Trainer Retention

The nature of the business is that trainers come and go. So, the goal is to keep them as long as you can, right? How do you do that?

Manager on Duty

My first boss in the fitness industry gave me some great advice. He said, *"You will always be on stage as a manager."* In other words, people are watching you everywhere you go, even when you hide in your office.

Do not hide in your office, or you will lose your trainers!

This is one of the main reasons gym owners or managers lose trainers; they become disconnected from them eventually — or worse, right from the start. The more you are out of your office educating, motivating, or monitoring your department, the more that staff member will think you care.

Incentive Programs

Money, more money and more money — the goal of all. The best motivator to get more money is money itself. As an owner, money comes on the front end and the back end of deals; you know this. So, if you give an incentive with trainer cash for new training sales and membership sales, the house wins in the end with membership dues. Money is the king when motivating trainers.

Part 2
From the Fitness Trainer's Point of View

"Think Win-Win!"

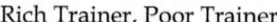

Win-Win will get you ahead every time!

40
Win-Win Thinking

Most fitness trainers either have too high expectations going into a job at a facility, or they don't live up to the owner's expectations. In order for a trainer to prosper, he or she must understand the environment and what limits that environment will have on him or her in the end.

If you are going to thrive and not just survive as a trainer who is employed by a gym owner, you will in the end have to come up with a *win-win* attitude and system.

High Expectations

Clients, clients, clients! That's all you ask for, right? Just give me clients, and I will stay out of your hair. This seems to be a trainer's mentality when he or she starts working in a gym. For whatever reason, you think that now that you are an employee of the facility, they should just supply you with income no matter what. Sorry, wrong—a good attitude to be fired by, maybe. With anything there are trade-offs, and you have to be realistic in each environment.

It's better to be surprised at your opportunities than to be let down by the lack thereof. I'm not telling you to temper your dreams and goals; just be aware of where the ceiling is.

In reality, there is only so much that a gym owner can do for you; the rest is up to you and how far you will meet him or her in the middle to better serve both you and the facility.

Bend, but Don't Break

In football, a popular style of defense is called *"Bend, but don't break."*

It means give a little but don't compromise your overall game plan or sell the farm.

If you work in a gym, there are trade-offs. You will eventually have to compromise somewhat to get the opportunity to stay employed there.

Trade-offs for Clients and Facility

Freedom! Some of your freedom is lost. You will not be able to control your schedule or fees; the house will determine that. Usually, though, the gym will give you a little freedom with a few things, but both of you have to have structure to make money.

There is no price for on-the-job training!

XI
Trainer Dude 100
"Things I Did Not Learn in the Classroom"

Trainer Dude 100 Overview

There is no better education than hands-on experience. There are no substitutes for it, either. Neither a piece of paper nor a person can just give it to you. You earn it by getting up in the morning, following your dreams, and striving toward a purpose. More often than not, true learning comes not in comforting times, but in challenging ones.

Today, fitness trainers make the vital mistake of hiding behind their accomplishments in the classroom, thinking that that's all there is to it and they will become successful. News flash: Not even close to the truth! Success is not in the X's and O's of a chart, but in the people themselves.

Trainer Dude 100 is a collection of things that I have observed and learned from the *"Real"* world through sweat, time, and my very own mistakes. This may be the most important book of the series, so I advise you to listen and take heed to every statement put forth in this book. **It WILL be the difference between you being *Rich* or *Poor* in the fitness training business.**

Do not make your profession in the fitness world complicated; it's not. Don't think that you have arrived at any point in your career, because that will be the beginning of the end for you. Do, however, compete only with yourself; fuel the creativity inside. Never fall prey to small-minded thinking on the outside, and love people for who they are, not what you want them to become.

Greg Ryan

Introduction

There is no better education than hands-on experience. There are no substitutes for it, either. Neither a piece of paper nor a person can just give it to you. You earn it by getting up in the morning, following your dreams, and striving toward a purpose. More often than not, true learning comes not in comforting times but in the challenging ones.

The fitness training business is a learning experience daily. One day you may learn something about a client; another time it could be about the profession itself. Then there are those times you learn hard lessons about yourself. Regardless, every situation is archived into your own little library of memories to be avoided or built upon at later times in your life.

The adventurous part of the fitness training business is that you will never learn everything. Some think that they have, but in the end are swallowed up by their own pride. Fitness training as a business takes mental flexibility and fortitude. Sure, there are medical guidelines to follow, but in the end it's about people and foresight, not charts, graphs or immediate gratification. Just surviving as a fitness trainer is challenging enough, but being successful year after year takes something special, and it takes working smart every single day.

My goal within these pages is to give you a little taste of what I have learned through my very own day-to-day experiences over the past thirty years. Conducting close to one hundred thousand hours of fitness training sessions, you can't help but learn a few valuable things about people's behaviors and needs, the business itself and what makes you tick, as well.

The statements or rules are in no order of importance based on their numbers; however, I guess you could say that they are ALL are important in their own application.

Be careful as you read these hundred or so little quotes and explanations. There are a lot of important things to learn between the lines. However, they are only as good as your implementation into your own life, career and business.

The "X" Factor
"The Gift"

A RICH fitness trainer and a POOR one are separated by two things: How they think, and how they use what God has given them. It sounds simple, but if that were the case, why aren't there more successful fitness trainers or coaches?

You've got to have something extra, know and care for people, use common sense and set up the right business template. RICH trainers have a quality that cannot be taught; it is what I call the **"X" Factor.** In other words, you need to be the Simon Cowell of fitness.

Here are a few things I learned about the importance of the "X" factor.

1. **Find your "Gift," harness it and ride the wave for the rest of your life.**

Each person has something that he or she is good at. Discover what it is, and apply it daily.

2. **Be careful how you think; small-town thinking will cost you dreams and cash.**

Believe in bigger things, not what others tell you to do.

3. **Your income is in direct relation to your self-worth.**

If you believe you can or can't, the outcome will be the same.

4. **Simplicity goes a long way, and makes you more money with less effort in the end.**

Don't complicate your career, people or your training methods; keep it real and simple.

5. Nurture creativity and snuff out competitiveness.
Constantly be imaginative and flexible, and avoid competing with others. Focus on a better you.

6. Love it or leave it!

No matter the money or the prestige, if you resent getting out of bed for work, don't. Love your job or leave it!

7. Love yourself, and respect your profession.

Care deeply for your well-being without ego; never think that you are above reproach.

8. Give to get

Before you can receive anything, you have to be willing to give it away — time, generosity, money, energy.

9. It's not about the money.

If you are a fitness trainer just to make money, you will NEVER be successful.

10. There are no options!

When times get tough, remember that there are no options but to move forward.

Business 101
"Sold Out"

Personal or fitness training is a *"business."* Attitudes, philosophies, principles, structure, policies and goals all must be a part of the developmental planning of that business. You are either sold out to your career or you're not, but that's just the start. Long-term, you are only as good as those you surround yourself with and how well you implement your business principles. Here are a few things pertaining to the business aspect of training that I have learned.

11. *"Lifers"* make more money than *"Part-timers."*

Have a *"Sold Out,"* attitude about your career and business from the beginning. And yes, it is a business!!

12. Freedom comes with a price, but when you get it, it's priceless.

Eventually, the only way to prosperity is to work for yourself.

13. Be *"Great"* at little rather than mediocre with a lot.

Find a niche, and be good at it. Don't complicate or dilute for the sake of ego.

14. Slave to the Lender — Avoid Bad Debt!

Avoid bad debt at all costs. Burdens cost money and squelch creativity.

15. Embrace "OJT" (On-the-Job-Training), and nurture Ph.D. or Education.

Classroom education is a must, but experience is the real teacher.

16. Develop *"Gatekeepers"* to protect your business interests.

Surround your business with quality business-minded people.

17. Do not get above your business.

Humility is the key to prosperity; ego is the brother of poverty.

18. Pillow talk is a disease of the mind and heart, and your business will die of a slow, hidden death.

Avoid personal relationships with employees, clients or business associates.

19. Business success is not based on numbers; it's gauged by longevity.

Concentrate on keeping your clients more than trying to get new ones — energy and money better spent.

20. Accountability is more important than compromise.

Establishing boundaries, enforcing business policies and holding people to their goals is more rewarding and cash-generating in the end than negotiating your principles.

Trainer Ethics 101
"Doing the Right Thing"

How you conduct your fitness training career is your business. Understand, though, that life will have its say, sooner or later. The success of your business is up to you, not your clients; how you go about getting it may be more important than the wealth, status or experience that you want to acquire.

Ethics, by definition, are moral principles you have inside you. Your actions, at their core, are determined by such morals, and life will either reward you for them or turn on you because of them. Your ethical beliefs affect yourself, others and your profession as a whole—remember that.

Each day you will have to decide: Follow what is right, even when it may not be popular, or compromise everything for the sake of the moment or circumstances. We live and die by our daily decisions. Here are some ethical standards to live by.

21. Let your actions speak so loudly that when you talk, they cannot hear you.

Make sure that your actions align with what you believe in and how you are acting.

22. If it's not popular with others in your profession, chances are it's the right thing to do.

Do the right thing even if it's not popular or the norm of those trainers around you.

23. The truth about Karma: It's real.

Do not undercut, backstab or talk about another trainer or fitness profession; it will only make you and the profession look and feel bad.

24. Say what you mean, and mean what you say.

Political correctness in the fitness business is an enabler.

25. One bad apple spoils the bunch.

Don't cast a bad light on an already disrespected profession by acting in an unethical way.

26. Avoid being a *"Wolf Spider"* at all costs.

Wolf Spiders eat their own. Do not talk about other trainers or bad-mouth them to others. It will only come back to bite you.

27. Dishonesty brings strife and poverty to your heart and business.

No matter what, tell your clients the truth; you owe them at least that. Your increase in income will show.

Psychology 101
"Free Your Mind"

Psychology is a vital part of the process within yourself. Competition comes not from the world as much as it does from within.

We control our lives and career by our thoughts and beliefs. Creativity and gratitude are the cornerstones of success, both emotionally and financially. Here are a few tips to think about when managing your own mind and fitness career.

28. A busy mind is the center of an unaccomplished career.

Practice quiet or meditation time; clients and money will then knock at your door.

29. Think creatively, and avoid competing.

Imagination attracts money, while competitive thinking or being concerned about another repels it.

30. You receive what you believe you are worth.

Your income is in direct relationship to how much confidence you have in your abilities.

31. You do not have because you do not ask.

Don't be afraid to ask for business.

32. The mind's eye does NOT know right from wrong.

Never underestimate the power of visualizing your business, future and income.

33. If you want money, be grateful for what you have first.

Gratitude is the key to open the door to the bank vault.

34. Your "Will" controls your pocketbook.

Believe it or not, you can "Will" things into existence, if you are strong enough to do the emotional work.

35. Free your mind, and the rest will follow.

Your mind is your biggest competitor — not life, other trainers or the economy. Free it up, and watch what happens.

Common Sense 101
"The Price of Ignorance"

Common sense is not learned or given as a gift; you either possess it, or you don't. Practicing good judgment in your business is as important as exercising is to losing weight.

When dealing with people, your business, or the profession, incorporating a common-sense approach to things is best. It's important to understand that it will take you twice as long and much more energy and money to succeed without it, assuming that you do. Here are a few common-sense things I have learned about fitness training.

36. Ignorance is the absence of common sense.

Without having a common-sense approach to your business, you will most likely not see failure coming.

37. Ego is a money stealer; humility is a money giver.

Your ego will cost you more money than anything else in your career.

38. "Storytell" for money.

If people can relate to a story, then you've got them emotionally connected. Common sense is sometimes in the form of a story.

39. Common sense may cost you a few cents.

Practicing good judgment in your business may cost you a penny in the beginning, but in the end will allow you to have more cents.

40. Lack of common sense sank the *Titanic*.

If you think that you are above reproach or your business is better than the rest, your business (ship) is already sinking — it's only a matter of time.

People 101
"EQ vs. "IQ"

Success is measured in relationships, not numbers. People are attracted to caring more than knowing. EQ reaches hearts more than IQ.

Every person is different, so your approach must be, as well. Master the *"Art"* of people, and the cash will be there for the taking. Here are some people skills and thoughts.

41. Relationships equal retention.

Invest in developing professional relationships with clients, and the financial payoff will be long-term.

42. EQ is more important and lucrative than IQ.

Motivating people is more emotional than intellectual. Learn about people, and the X's and O's are easy.

43. One size does not fit all.

One type of exercise approach does not work for everyone. You have to address personality types to succeed.

44. Give responsibility, and expect accountability.

People feel better about themselves when accomplishing things or assignments; however, sometimes they need to be made to do so.

45. Train based on personality.

Two types of personalities need two different approaches.

46. Assumptions are expensive.

Do not make assumptions about people's income, likeness of you, buying power or commitment level.

47. Give people what they NEED, not what they want.

Hold people accountable to their goals; they WANT that.

48. People don't expect you to know everything, but they do expect honesty.

Admit when you may not know an answer — be honest ALL of the time.

EQ is more lucrative than IQ.

Leadership 101
"Lead with Silence"

Being a good leader requires guts, a spine and faith. In the fitness business, you are paid to lead, no matter what. Holding an adult in this world accountable for his or her actions goes against the grain, and at times is not politically correct. So, what? Leaders are lonely at the top by nature. Lead or follow — that's your choice. Here are few leadership things to ponder.

49. No guts, no glory.

Leadership requires confidence; confidence makes money.

50. Empty words are like getting free advice — and then they send you the bill.

Don't be a hypocrite. Through your actions, make your words have weight behind them.

51. Honesty and transparency build cash bridges.

If you don't know an answer, say you don't, and find it out. People know when you are "B.S.-ing" them.

52. Leading sometimes means NOT leading.

Leaders learn to say no when need be. If you are a yes person, you are a poor one, too.

53. Lead by sometimes doing the opposite.

Stick with YOUR plan, even if it means sometimes going against the grain of your peers.

54. Lead by empowering, not degrading.

Inspiration with accountability and love is always more profitable than with degradation and fear.

Marketing 101
"Leveraging Your Brand"

Marketing and branding are necessities in the fitness training business. Work smart or waste cash—not easy to predetermine. The art is in the leveraging. The power is in your brand. Like a lot of things, it's not rocket science, but it does require discipline, dedication and perseverance.

The key is to not forget the best way of building relationships, while at the same time not being left behind in today's social media world and technology. Here are a few tips that I've learned.

55. Either you stand for something, or you fall for anything.

Making a name means being the same person all the time. Decide your identity, and never deviate.

56. Never deface your logo.

Once it's out there, never add to your logo; it lessens the power of your brand by confusing the market.

Branding says nothing without leverage.

57. Branding is about consistency, not hard-selling.

When creating a name for yourself, focus on being consistent with something more than in-your-face selling.

58. Without trust, marketing means nothing.

No matter how you market your brand, you have to consistently build trust between you and your clients.

59. Personal and Social go together in today's world.

You will not succeed as a fitness trainer today without marketing with social media and building personal face-to-face relationships.

60. Good marketers build a following through education, not sales promotions.

Building a group of followers today is about consistently educating, not selling them.

K.I.S.S.
Keep it simple!

Nutrition 101
"Big Picture"

Dealing with food is an "Attitude" as much as it is counting calories; maybe even more so. You always have to look at food from the big-picture perspective.

Keeping the big picture in mind does not mean that you have to be a dietitian. You can educate and encourage, while at the same time not confusing or complicating things. A fitness trainer's purpose is more in the follow-through than in the food itself. Leave the hard stuff to someone else. Here are some things to chew on when implementing nutrition advice in your business.

70. Chose your battles carefully.

You are not a dietitian; don't claim to be.

71. Food and fitness are more about accountability than calorie counting.

A trainer's job is more about encouraging awareness of eating habits than solving the X's and O's.

72. Playing psychologist and therapist is part of the job.

Changing eating habits is about discovering emotional attachments to food and changing them.

73. Emotional accountability is physically harder than any exercise responsibility.

Holding people accountable to good eating habits at home takes emotional confidence, more so than making then run.

74. Push too hard, and deprivation steps in; encourage too little, and perseverance gives in.

Changing one's food habits is a long process. With too many boundaries, people rebel; with not enough guidelines, they lose hope and confidence.

75. Play the percentages.

Do not get too hung up on micromanaging; help your clients learn the percentages of types of foods—not always a calorie issue.

Gym Owner - Fitness Director 101
"Motivate for More Money"

The goal: increase cash flow and decrease turnover. Owners and directors seek fairness and balance with fitness trainers. Here are a few things to think about in managing this part of your business:

76. Complacency breeds poverty.

Gym owners, managers or directors should never lose touch with their staff by hiding in their office.

77. Cultivate relationships with honesty.

Map out in writing all of your businesses guidelines and policies. Make sure that they understand in writing what is expected of them.

78. Creativity spawns cash flow.

Be open and get your trainers involved in creating incentive programs for themselves. Who said you have to do the industry norm?

Decrease Turnover – Increase Cash Flow

79. Consistency pays

Whatever trainer policy you implement, do it consistently with ALL trainers. Favors undermine your authority.

80. CYA

Cover your butt. Always require liability insurance. At the very least, it builds respect between you and the trainer.

81. Clothing *not* optional

Depending on your trainer policy, it's always best to have a dress code.

82. Cash flow by committee

Create a manager-on-duty program, with one person in charge of the floor for a period of time. Confidence creates cash.

83. Confine and conquer

Confine all drama and disputes to each individual. Conquer it before it gets out of control and you lose control.

The money is in the "Art!"

The "Art" of Fitness Training 101

Fitness training is an *"Art"* as much as it is a profession. If you are fortunate to get results consistently, you may survive. After thirty years, I have been blessed to have built a small fortune because I have never forgotten the little things during a client training session that make all the world of difference in their success and mine in the end.

It's not rocket science, but you have to — even for a session — take your mind off of yourself and put yourself in the shoes of the other person. Here are a few training session tips that have made me a million that you should ALWAYS do.

84. Tuck your shirt in.

Always look like a professional and act like one. Branding is everything.

85. Timing is everything.

Be on time, no matter what, even if they are not.

86. Accessorize with less.

No phones, coffee cups, TV or people watching.

87. Accountability is the key to cash.

Enforce payment, session and scheduling policies.

88. Obey the "One-Way" rule.

Trainers are paid to listen, not share personal information.

89. Sleeping with the enemy.

Absolutely no sexual relationships with clients. The "Well" will go dry.

90. Keep your hand on the pulse.

Always monitor heart rates during workout sessions.

91. Respect the "All or Nothing" rule.

Educate and motivate clients on all components of wellness; do not piecemeal your sessions with just weights.

92. Follow up for cash.

Never allow 48 hours between connecting with a current client. This helps client retention.

93. Never be afraid to say no.

If you don't know an answer to a question, say you don't; then, within twenty-four hours, get it.

94. Motivate by being methodical.

If possible, do not go by a clock to stop your sessions. Be fluid, set a good pace, and get as much accomplished as possible.

95. Enforce the "Technology-Free" Zone.

Unless it's an emergency, do not allow phone calls, either by the client or you.

96. No shoes, no service.

Not only for safety's sake, but to also to send a message about being serious—if they forget their shoes, no session.

97. Ride the "Ten-Week Wave," and then get off.

If you have a set routine for a client, change it up around the ten-week mark. Anything more breeds stagnation.

98. Testing for Retention

Periodic fitness testing around every six to eight weeks better ensures that your clients will stick with you.

99. Empty words equal empty wallets.

If at all possible, do not coach someone to do something that you are not willing to do or have done; these are words without meaning to clients.

100. A joyful trainer is a RICH TRAINER.

Whatever you do, enjoy your work. When you don't, it's time to do something else.

I would not take a million bucks for the "On-the-Job Training" or "OJT" experience I have received over the last three decades. My classroom education got me started, but the real world taught me to keep going. The fact is, neither you nor I will learn everything there is to know; each day will be a new learning experience.

What I have discovered is that you will definitely learn about yourself and what you're made of. OJT will mold you, define you and educate you on the REAL world. **Fitness training is a people business more so than a numbers game. It requires more emotions and creativity than logic or reason; understand this, and you will be RICH; neglect it, and stay POOR.**

Remember, it's the little things that matter most in customer care. At the same time, it's the big picture that's most important when taking care of your business.

Never lose your joy while in the trenches. No matter how dirty it may get, lose your reasons and lose your soul. Be a trainer to empower and inspire, not for finances or fame; true intentions build longevity.

Conclusion

Yes, this is only the beginning! Conclusions usually mean tying things up or the end of something. For you and me, however, let's look at this as the beginning to a new way of thinking with our fitness career.

At the end of the day, there might be no difference between you or me, at least on a physical level. However, mentally we can be worlds apart, separated by the space between our ears. You want to be RICH in this business? Think it first; believe it second. Make it a profession, and never get above reproach. Learn people from the inside out, encourage when wanted, and hold accountable when needed. Surround yourself with good-character people telling you the truth in love; be grateful for everything, and remember that you are your biggest competitor, not others.

You get what you think and give. You attract into your business what you believe to be your truth. Pay attention to detail, yet manage from afar. Do this, and you are already wealthy. Treat people well and do what you love, and you will be happy.

My best,

Greg Ryan

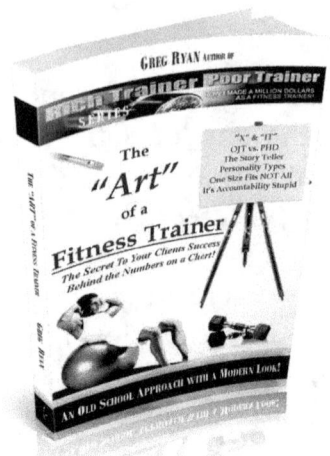

The *"Art"* of a Fitness Trainer
The Secrets to Your Clients' Success Behind the Numbers on the Charts!

The "Art" of a Fitness Trainer book is about the client and trainer's workout session. When training clients, it's not all about educating them on X's and O's on a chart. Sure, that's the nuts and bolts, but there are few little things that you can do to keep them longer as clients, and let's be real: The goal is retention—how long they stay!

TEN SECRETS TO KEEPING YOUR CLIENTS
5 YEARS OR MORE!

ON SALE NOW AT AMAZON!

RICH TRAINER, POOR TRAINER

For more information, you may go to **www.rich-trainer.com** or e-mail us at **greg@resolutions.bz**.

Follow us on twitter at Richtrainer1 or Rich Trainer on Facebook.

Greg Ryan's Other Companies:

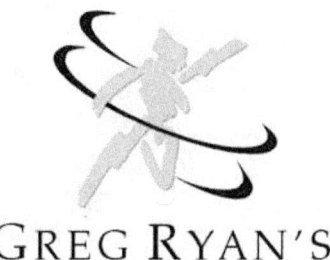

GREG RYAN'S
Elite Training and Weight Loss Systems

Tel: 502.295.8555   **Email: greg@resolutions.bz**

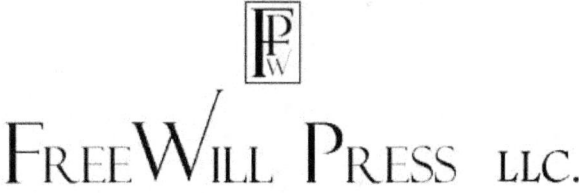

FREEWILL PRESS LLC.
Book Publishing ~ Public Speaking ~ Life Coaching!

Greg Ryan CEO

What's Your Story?   Tel.502.295.8555